DISABILITY POLITICS AND CARE

Christine Kelly

DISABILITY POLITICS AND CARE

The Challenge of Direct Funding

UBCPress · Vancouver · Toronto

24 23 22 21 20 19 18 17 16   5 4 3 2 1

Printed in Canada on FSC-certified ancient-forest-free paper (100% post-consumer recycled) that is processed chlorine- and acid-free.

Library and Archives Canada Cataloguing in Publication

Kelly, Christine, author
    Disability politics and care : the challenge of Direct Funding / Christine Kelly.

Includes bibliographical references and index.
Issued in print and electronic formats.
ISBN 978-0-7748-3009-6 (bound). – ISBN 978-0-7748-3011-9 (pdf). –
ISBN 978-0-7748-3012-6 (epub). – ISBN 978-0-7748-3013-3 (mobi)

    1. Direct Funding Program. 2. People with disabilities – Care – Ontario. 3. People with disabilities – Services for – Ontario. 4. People with disabilities – Government policy – Ontario. I. Title.

HV1559.C3K44 2016   362.409713   C2015-903886-3
                                                              C2015-903887-1

Canadä

UBC Press gratefully acknowledges the financial support for our publishing program of the Government of Canada (through the Canada Book Fund), the Canada Council for the Arts, and the British Columbia Arts Council.

This book has been published with the help of a grant from the Canadian Federation for the Humanities and Social Sciences, through the Awards to Scholarly Publications Program, using funds provided by the Social Sciences and Humanities Research Council of Canada.

A reasonable attempt has been made to secure permission to reproduce all material used. If there are errors or omissions they are wholly unintentional and the publisher would be grateful to learn of them.

Printed and bound in Canada by Friesens
Set in Myriad and Minion by Artegraphica Design Co. Ltd.
Copy editor: Judy Phillips
Proofreader: Sophie Pouyanne
Indexer: Judy Dunlop

UBC Press
The University of British Columbia
2029 West Mall
Vancouver, BC V6T 1Z2
www.ubcpress.ca

This book is dedicated to Dale and Ian,
and to all the disability activists, artists, and scholars
who make it possible to imagine and to live
disability differently.

Contents

Acknowledgments

A sole-authored book contributes to the myth of independence and the exaltation of autonomy, suggesting that an individual can participate in the world without support. Acknowledgments help to counter these myths, and there are many people who influenced the content of these pages.

The book would not be possible without the considerable donation of time and ideas from the people with disabilities, attendants, informal supports, and key informants who participated in qualitative interviews, with only coffee, chocolate, or cookies for compensation. We met at their homes, their workplaces, and in coffee shops, and all who participated were generous with their time, insights, and ideas. "Killian," in particular, went above and beyond the interviews to play an important role in this project and continues to be a loyal friend. Thank you sincerely for your willingness to tell your stories.

This project had its genesis at Carleton University, and it is essential to acknowledge the thoughtful contributions and encouragement from Hugh Armstrong. Conversations with, and feedback from, Hugh helped to nuance my exploration of feminist care scholarship, and I am honoured to have worked so closely with such a prolific and widely regarded researcher. I am greatly indebted to Pauline Rankin, and it is difficult to describe the extent of her influence on me. Pauline is generous with her time and met with me throughout (and after) my time at Carleton. Pauline shared her thoughts and observations on matters big and small, and continues to be an important figure in and beyond my scholarship. Roy Hanes served as a commendable example of "practicing alliance" throughout his career, reminding me of the importance of being both accountable to, and involved with, disability communities. Sally Chivers's attention to detail and positive comments were always encouraging. Christina Gabriel and Michelle Owen also provided invaluable feedback to this work.

I must also acknowledge the support from my colleagues at the University of Ottawa as this project evolved into a book. Shoshana Magnet graciously shared an example of a book proposal when we had just met. Michael Orsini is an attentive and sensitive colleague, willing to contribute in a multitude of ways to my work. Michael is up to date with the latest developments on all my projects, always ready with a solution, empathetic ear, or joke. I am grateful for his ongoing support and friendship. Emily Andrew from UBC Press has been a dedicated editor, providing guidance and demonstrating patience during a long discussion of book titles. The entire UBC Press team has been wonderful in moving the manuscript to production. The anonymous reviewers of the manuscript provided feedback that strengthened the final manuscript in substantial ways.

In the background of this history is a lively network of disability-studies colleagues in Canada and beyond. Like many in academia, I found myself reading and exploring disability on my own but making connections with others online and in-person at conferences. The social media updates, discussions at conferences, and writing of my colleagues in disability studies have been essential to the formation of my ideas. The words, in no particular order, of Tanya Titchkosky, Rod Michalko, Anne McGuire, Kelly Fritsch, Katie Aubrecht, Eliza Chandler, Jay Dolmage, Patty Douglas, Chris Chapman, Jihan Abbas, Deborah Stienstra, Nancy Hansen, Katherine Runswick-Cole, Jenny Slater, Rebecca Mallett, Nirmala Erevelles, Leslie Freeman, Jeff Preston, Mary Jean Hande, Sam Walsh, jes sachse, Nancy Halifax, and many others echo through these pages.

On a more practical basis, the graduate scholarships from the Social Sciences and Humanities Research Council, the Banting Postdoctoral fellowship program, Awards to Scholarly Publications Program, and internal research funding from the University of Ottawa gave the material means and space to do this work. The Publication Grant through the Awards to Scholarly Publications Program was particularly important; this program is essential to the flourishing of Canadian-based scholarship.

I want to acknowledge the under-recognized care work that makes it possible for me to participate in higher education, namely the frequent visits and support from my parents, Michelle and Herb, and my mother-in-law, Joan. I must also acknowledge the work of our dedicated daycare provider, Brianna

Bowman, who takes very good care of our distracting toddler, Ian. Thanks to our friend Kevin Morrissey, who helps out in the evenings when I am not available, and did so even when Ian was very young. And, of course, I want to acknowledge the steady support from Dale, who creates community with disabled people everywhere he goes, is deeply moved by the participants' words shared in these pages, and is a motivating force for my scholarship.

Previously Published Material

A version of Chapter 1 was previously published by John Wiley and Sons as

Kelly, Christine. 2013. "Building Bridges with Accessible Care: Disability Studies, Feminist Care Scholarship and Beyond." *Hypatia* 28 (4): 784–800.

A version of Chapter 4 was previously published by Oxford University Press as

Kelly, Christine. 2014. "Re/moving Care from the Ontario Direct Funding Program: Altering Conversations among Disability and Feminist Scholars." *Social Politics: International Studies in Gender, State & Society* 21 (1): 124–47.

DISABILITY POLITICS AND CARE

Introduction
The Tensions of Care

Jennifer has lived in an array of long-term care settings in Ontario, including in a hospital-like residential centre, where she was institutionalized as a child, and presently in her own home, where she receives cash to directly hire attendants to support her. This range of experiences shapes Jennifer's political views and gives her a unique perspective from which to comment on long-term care for people with disabilities in Ontario. When describing the residential centre from her childhood, Jennifer explained that the staff members knew each of the fifty-two children with physical disabilities who lived there, yet they decided to institute hospital bracelets for identification. Jennifer and the other children resisted the bracelets, seeing them as impractical and demeaning, but the staff insisted they were necessary. Jennifer recounts:

> We cut them off. And the kids who couldn't cut it off themselves, we helped them cut it off. And kids would chew them off. Every day they were replacing these bracelets with us. They just gave up. So we wore them down. We won that battle.

Jennifer and the other children resented the bracelets that stood for the medicalization of their bodies and the complete control of their lives, and literally chewed them off their bodies to make a dramatic statement about life in a large institution.

"I offer an apology to the men, women and children of Ontario who were failed by a model of institutional care for people with developmental disabilities."

In December 2013, Ontario premier Kathleen Wynne delivered this historic public apology, acknowledging the harms and "deeply flawed" approach of government-funded regional centres for people with developmental disabilities, which ran in parallel to the hospitals for children with physical disabilities, such as the one where Jennifer lived as a child.[1] The litany of harms include physical, emotional, and sexual abuse; ineffective "therapies"; human degradation through social isolation; and complete control over the lives of individuals who lived in the centres, all of which took place under the guise of "care" for disabled populations. The premier characterized the regional centres as a painful chapter in the history of the province of Ontario. This apology followed the closing of all regional centres in 2009, and was part of a class-action settlement against the Ontario government led by former residents.

Mass institutionalization of disabled people, like other forms of systematic oppression, cannot be contained to a specific historic period. The harms, abuses, and human degradation associated with social segregation and the material effects of this exclusion continue to haunt institutional survivors and their families and friends, as well as, more broadly, people with disabilities who do not have direct experience living in institutions. Models of institutional care continue to structure other care arrangements for people with all types of impairments, even if services are delivered in smaller settings that are designed to be home-like and endorse community-oriented frameworks. Paternalistic and "caring" approaches to disability pervade popular perceptions and shape individual encounters between nondisabled and disabled people. In short, this history is not a history. The effects of these models of care cannot be erased by glossing over or tangibly repurposing former institutional sites (Abbas and Voronka 2014).

Jennifer also recounted challenges she faced in every single support arrangement that she lived in over the years after leaving the residential centre, many

---

[1] Many authors explore questions of terminology in their work on disability (e.g., Shakespeare 2006; Siebers 2008; Titchkosky 2003). These discussions explore the extent to which disability is socially constructed, the power of naming, and whether disability is central or marginal to personal identity. There are some regional and generational elements to this discussion, that is, generally people in the United Kingdom and people coming from a cultural framework use the term "disabled people," whereas some people in North America and established leaders tend to use "people with disabilities." In my experience, this debate also occurs in disability-related organizations and among individuals with disabilities, including participants in this study (see also Watson 2002). Since there is no consensus regionally, within disability movements, or within academia, I use both of the most widely accepted terms, that is, "people with disabilities" and "disabled people."

of which were positioned as alternatives to medical, institutional, and caring approaches to disability. She reflects, "Wherever they are, people want choice. They want autonomy, they want more control over where they are." Lack of choice over major and minor life decisions, from relationships and employment to what to wear and eat, is one of the most pervasive and perhaps subtle violences of institutionalization. Enabling choice for all disabled people became the crux of Jennifer's activism over her lifetime and reflects the broader framework of the Independent Living movement.

The recent history of mass institutionalization, the caring mentalities and attitudes that continue to undergird support for people with disabilities, and the political efforts to contain institutionalization to a specific historic period all forge a difficult backdrop for present-day attendant services. Part of this challenge is to bring the critiques of institutional care to the many researchers, practitioners, activists, and students from varied backgrounds who work in care-related fields. Care is arguably a foundational orientation and pivotal goal of many health and social sciences fields and policy discussions and, for many, a motivating force for the work they do. To complicate things further, "care" is a common word, often deployed in business names and mandates, extending far beyond the worlds of disability movements and health and social policies. The ubiquitous presence of care, however, does not imply a lack of controversy, as demonstrated by both Jennifer's life story and the apology from Premier Wynne.

Independent Living movements, disability activists, and disabled individuals worldwide proclaim, "We do not need care." This statement comes from even those with profound physical and intellectual impairments, some of whom require comprehensive, ongoing assistance with daily activities that might otherwise be described as care. Disability movements do not intend to eliminate the provision of daily physical assistance, so which meanings and practices of care *are* rejected in this sentiment? *Disability Politics and Care* aims to interrogate the foundational concept of care and to consider the implications of taking seriously the rejection of care presented by disability movements and individuals with disabilities. That is, the book explores what it might mean to acknowledge the disability critiques and to incorporate a rejection of care into the core of theorizing, research, practices, and policies of care.

The central objective of *Disability Politics and Care* is thus to document contemporary practices and conceptualizations of care within a program that explicitly rejects it: Ontario's Direct Funding Program, the same program Jennifer uses. The program is administered by a nonprofit organization affiliated with international Independent Living movements. Independent Living has a vibrant history that includes rejecting caring approaches to disability while redefining independence. Independent Living is a (sometimes) effective social and political placeholder that offers valuable commentary on care. It is also a fragile social movement managing to survive in hostile neoliberal and austerity policy climates. Academic debates about care build on Independent Living critiques, and occur most often and directly between disability scholars and activists on the one hand, and feminist care researchers aiming to revalue gendered forms of labour on the other. Rather than seeking common ground between the disability and feminist perspectives, this book instead defines care as a tension. I argue that the tensions and competing meanings are integral to common, and uncommon, understandings of care.

Disability Politics and Care considers this tension from the perspectives of the individuals at the centre of the debates – that is, through reporting on fifty-four qualitative, in-depth interviews with people with disabilities, attendants, informal supports, and key informants from varied sectors related to Ontario's Direct Funding Program. Through these conversations, I found that direct-funding mechanisms and the connections to disability movements rhetorically remove care but do not eliminate it. Rather, care is moved and contained to specific meanings, transforming our understandings and practices in the process. I term this process "removing care" or the "removal of care." *Disability Politics and Care* has implications that extend beyond the specific program to resonate in parallel policy spheres and throughout Canadian and international disability movements.

The tensions of care and the related academic debates take place in the context of attendant services for people with disabilities. According to the Attendant Services Advisory Committee (ASAC), attendant services primarily serve people with physical disabilities. As ASAC describes: "Consumers direct their attendants to perform the activities of daily living (ADL) they require to get on with their day-to-day lives. Attendant services include: bathing and washing, transferring, toileting, dressing, skin care, essential communications, and meal preparation. The consumer is responsible for the decisions and training involved in his/her own services" (OCSA 2008).[2] Attendant services can also include help with cleaning, household maintenance, errands, and

---

[2] In material influenced by Independent Living philosophy, people with disabilities are commonly referred to as "consumers" in an effort to position disability-related programs as services and disabled people in charge of these services. There are issues with this term and ongoing discussions in the community about it. "Consumer" makes concessions to a mass-produced culture, may overvalue individualism and choice, and implies options when none may be available. Thus, because of these debates and since it is less widely used than the phrases discussed in the preceding note, I do not use this term other than in a direct quotation.

sometimes child care. Attendant services are rooted in the Independent Living movement and are premised on the notion of consumer direction, which shifts control of the services to people with disabilities. Attendant services influenced by Independent Living often include an explicit rejection of the concept of care. Language is a primary indicator of this approach and is reflected not only in the aversion to the term "care" but also in the choosing of terms such as "self-manager" and "consumer" when referring to people with disabilities using the services, and "attendant" (in Ontario) and "personal assistant" (most common in the United States and the United Kingdom) when referring to the person providing the service.[3]

Perhaps the culmination of Independent Living attendant services that is clearly linked to an adamant rejection of care is directly-funded service delivery.[4] "Direct funding" refers to providing public funds to disabled people, nonprofit organizations, and, in some cases, family members or guardians to hire individuals to provide assistance with daily needs. In direct-funding arrangements, people with disabilities become the employers (in varying respects) of their attendants and are often required to take on administrative duties previously in the purview of service-provision organizations or governments. Disability movements and related organizations pushed for this style of service delivery in the United Kingdom, in various US states, and throughout Canada because of the associated flexibility, empowerment, and user control it provides for disabled people (Mladenov 2012). The push for direct funding has transformed into advocacy and pilot programs for individualized or personalized budgets that expand the eligible activities beyond attendant services and aim to account for the diverse needs and services of a wider range of disabled people. There are sixteen documented direct-funding programs among the ten Canadian provinces (none in the territories or on First Nations reserves), plus an option through the Veterans Independence Program, a service of Veterans Affairs Canada (Spalding, Watkins, and Williams 2006). The Ontario version is the only Canadian example that was developed and piloted, and continues to be administered, by an Independent Living organization. Canada has a national network of Independent Living organizations with strong connections to disability movements in North America, and at times, this network is characterized as a movement itself (Lord 2010).

---

3 "Self-manager" is the term used in Ontario's Direct Funding Program materials and is used in this book.

4 The term "self-managed (home) care" has some currency in Canada, though "direct funding" is the most popular term in Ontario.

The Self-Managed Attendant Services in Ontario Direct Funding Program – known more simply as the Direct Funding Program – is administered by the Centre for Independent Living in Toronto (CILT). The program, piloted in 1995–96, was established as a permanent program in 1998 and is funded through the Ontario Ministry of Health and Long-Term Care (Parker et al. 2000). In 2011, when the study this book is based on was conducted, 676 people were using Direct Funding, out of the approximately 6,000 people who were documented in 2008 as using attendant services in Ontario (Katherine Janicki, Direct Funding clerk at CILT, pers. comm.; OCSA 2008). To demonstrate the relative size of attendant services and Direct Funding, Bannerjee (2009) documents 70,100 long-term care beds in Ontario in 2004; this number includes supportive housing (as does the 6,000 count) but does not include attendant outreach services or Direct Funding recipients.[5] Taking into consideration the ambiguity of the figures, the number of people using Direct Funding in Ontario makes up less than 1 percent of long-term care service users and roughly 11.6 percent of attendant-service users. This percentage is similar to direct-funding use elsewhere, with the exception of increases in the uptake of Direct Payments in the United Kingdom in the mid-2000s (Hall 2011).[6] Despite its small scope, the Ontario program is the largest direct-funding program in Canada in terms of the number of people assuming the full responsibilities of being an employer and receiving cash transfers (Spalding, Watkins, and Williams 2006). The program is by far the most independent model of attendant services in the Ontario landscape, and in 2011 had a four-year waiting list, with approximately four hundred people on it. In January 2014, Deb Matthews, the Ontario minister of Health and Long-Term Care, announced that the Direct Funding Program would receive an injection of capital that would enable approximately three hundred more people to become self-managers and reduce the waiting list from four years to two, signifying increased political support for this program (CILT 2014). In a broader context, the Ontario government will fund self-directed and directly funded home-care pilot projects for older Canadians in the fall of 2015. The cultural messages inextricably tied to the history and the current information on the Direct Funding Program declare that people with disabilities do not need

---

[5] Attendant outreach services are prescheduled, at-home/at-work personal support provided through Community Support Services. People with disabilities may be involved in the administration of these programs, but on a day-to-day basis, individuals using the program do not directly choose who will be supporting them and may have to compromise the time of service based on the needs of others using the program.

[6] Direct funding is known as "Direct Payments" in the United Kingdom.

care and can collectively and individually manage disability-related services. Access to quality attendant services is framed as a right that enables people with disabilities to fully participate in society, making the Direct Funding Program an interesting case study with which to explore care.

This book highlights the strengths of the program and makes tentative recommendations for improvements where appropriate; however, the primary aim is to enter into theoretical discussions of care. Specifically, this book enters into the debates and conversations between feminist care researchers and disability perspectives and explores the broader policy and movement effects of these discussions. The Direct Funding Program can be characterized as embracing a disability perspective that explicitly rejects the concept of care. As is discussed throughout *Disability Politics and Care*, there are wide-reaching implications of the messages conveyed through this small program. This argument begins by exploring the program within the context of social and political factors in Ontario. Considering the position of the Direct Funding Program among disability movements, the Ontario policy landscape, shifts in social policy and medicine, and globalized care patterns, it is clear that the program guidelines, those who administer it, and those who use it are remarkable examples of social movement activity in a highly constrained context.

Direct Funding among Disability Movements

Ontario's Direct Funding Program builds on numerous historical precedents and can be situated within disability movements in the United States, the United Kingdom, and Canada. Direct-funding models of support can be linked to the deinstitutionalization movement from the 1950s onwards, which seeks to transition people with disabilities and mental health concerns physically out of large-scale institutes and metaphorically out of institutionalized approaches to disability (Ben-Moshe, Chapman, and Carey 2014; Gardner and Glanville 2005; Stroman 2003). The ongoing deinstitutionalization movement is largely led by parent advocates, people with intellectual disabilities, and people with mental health concerns. As briefly mentioned at the outset of this chapter, in March 2009, Ontario closed the final three large-scale institutions, namely the Huronia Regional Centre, the Rideau Regional Centre, and the Southwestern Regional Centre. Institutionalized approaches, however, continue to structure the lives of many people with intellectual impairments living in group homes and long-term care homes throughout Ontario and other parts of Canada (Ben-Moshe, Chapman, and Carey 2014; Canadian Association for Community Living and People First of Canada 2011). Following the closures, former residents of the

Huronia Regional Centre, located in Orillia, Ontario, launched a class-action lawsuit alleging that the Ontario government "failed to properly care and protect the people who lived at Huronia" and "that residents of Huronia were emotionally, physically, and psychologically traumatized by their experiences at Huronia" (Crawford Class Action Services 2014). The suit resulted in a $35 million settlement for people who lived at the centre between 1945 and 2009 and a formal apology from Ontario premier Kathleen Wynne; it was then followed by two related settlements for former residents of the Rideau Regional Centre and the Southwestern Regional Centre (Institutional Survivors 2014; Ontario Ministry of Community and Social Services 2013). The historical and political significance of these settlements is a salient backdrop to the ongoing history of direct funding. Deinstitutionalization activities highlight the often deplorable living conditions in segregated residences, as well as the cultural messages about disability conveyed through social isolation, medicalization, lack of choice, routinization of life, and inhumane treatment. The deinstitutionalization movement demands that people with disabilities live in community settings, and the Direct Funding Program is a potential mechanism for making this possible. At least two participants in this study lived in large-scale institutions as children, reflecting strong links between the Direct Funding Program and deinstitutionalization. Unlike programs in five other provinces, the Ontario example does not serve people with intellectual disabilities or mental health issues unless a physical impairment is also present and the individual can demonstrate the ability to self-direct (Spalding, Watkins, and Williams 2006). The relationship of Direct Funding to intellectual disability is taken up throughout this book.

Elements of the social model of disability also resonate with the Direct Funding Program. As most commonly described, the social model refers to the concept articulated by Paul Hunt of the British organization Union of the Physically Impaired against Segregation in the early 1970s and refined with a materialist lens by Mike Oliver (1990). The social model argues that disability is a social construction: people are disabled primarily by societal structures and attitudes and not by their biological impairments (Campbell and Oliver 1996; K. Davis 1993). The social model is often cited as the basis for disability organizing in the United Kingdom (Campbell and Oliver 1996), though it has undergone substantive critique in academic spheres (e.g., Shakespeare and Watson 2002; Corker 1999) and does not exemplify the intricate theorizing and scholarship that now characterizes the field of disability studies. However, the more complex theoretical scholarship is not necessarily as accessible to, or visible within, community organizations and activist efforts related to disability (with some exceptions), whereas to an extent, the social model has managed to permeate common parlance in these arenas. Like the Direct Funding Program, the social model draws attention to the environment of disability and promotes the removal of barriers and the provision of supports in order to mediate the effects of impairments. As is found at a few points in this study, the availability of reliable, respectful, and sufficient attendant services makes living with a disability in an ableist society easier, and "mediates citizenship" by creating the conditions for diverse participation (Krogh 2004, 139).

Most significantly, the Direct Funding Program can be interpreted as the quintessential manifestation of the Independent Living movement. Direct-funding schemes build on the legacy of disability leader Ed Roberts and a group of students with disabilities who named themselves the Rolling Quads. In the 1970s, this group was forced to live in a hospital while attending the University of California, Berkeley, because of physically inaccessible residences. Initially, the Rolling Quads focused on living independently yet integrated in the community, and the group founded the first of many Independent Living centres in the United States (Longmore 2003). Like deinstitutionalization, Independent Living is a philosophical commitment. "Independent Living philosophy," as it is termed on websites and community newsletters, values disability as a social role, emphasizes rights discourse and consumer control, redefines independence in terms of decision making, and is a central orientation of many direct-funding programs.

Disability movements emerged in Canada in the early 1980s and can be distinguished from American and British movements in numerous ways. Scholars note that Canadian disability activists and organizations played an integral role in establishing an international disability rights movement (Driedger 1989) and have a long history within the nonprofit sector (Neufeldt 2003). These organizations and activists work closely with Canadian governments and are often characterized as employing nonconfrontational tactics (Chivers 2007; Valentine 1996). The Canadian Independent Living movement in particular has an emphasis on individual advocacy rather than on collective action, in contrast to the approach of its American counterparts (Lord 2010; Valentine 1994).

In many ways, Ontario's Direct Funding Program is a seamless fit with the goals, history, and approach of disability movements in North America and the United Kingdom – that is, it's a seamless fit with the movement histories that are well documented. Some of the most oft-cited historical events in Canada could be easily replaced by the Direct Funding history. For example, accounts of how people with disabilities garnered inclusion in the Canadian Charter of Rights and Freedoms (Peters 2003) present a seemingly unanimous, policy-focused, nonconfrontational, consultation-based achievement that resonates with the establishment of the Direct Funding Program. As is explored further in Chapter 6, there are other, less well-recorded elements and factions of Canadian disability organizing that do not fit as well.

Disability movements in the United Kingdom and the United States have also pushed for direct-funding models of service delivery, setting precedents for the Ontario example. Overwhelmingly, these programs are evaluated as highly successful, cost-effective, and empowering (Blyth and Gardner 2007; Caldwell and Heller 2007; Stainton and Boyce 2004; Carmichael and Brown 2002; Leece 2000; Askheim 1999), and this can be said of the Ontario example also (Parker et al. 2000; Roeher Institute 1997). In Ontario, community organizations and advocates participated in writing the policy and continue to administer the program, raising interesting questions for the future roles of disability movements (Yoshida et al. 2000). This may indicate that if individuals or disability organizations take issue with the administration of the program, they are in the uncomfortable situation of having to direct efforts at a fellow disability organization. Most of the advocacy of the program and attendant services more broadly is targeted at the Ontario Ministry of Health and Long-Term Care. For example, the Attendant Services Advisory Committee (which includes representatives from CILT) recommends attendant-service waiting lists be added to the Provincial Wait List Strategy, funding be increased to the sector, and additional individualizing funding options be made available (OCSA 2008). Also in Ontario, community advocate Scott Allardyce proposed draft legislation called the Consumer Attendant Support Services Protection Act, which would provide a venue for attendant service users to report abuse and includes recommendations for a consumer advocate office, reduced wait times, and mechanisms for dispute resolution (draft legislation; Scott Allardyce, pers. comm.). Citizens with Disabilities – Ontario (CWDO) formally declared support for Allardyce's proposed legislation, advocated that the Ontario Ministry of Health and Long-Term Care reduce the Direct Funding waiting list, and hosted webinars with practical advice on managing attendants. CWDO's position paper on attendant services also includes an explicit rejection of care. Indeed, most of the current advocacy of Direct Funding is consistent and cooperative, systems focused, and directed at the provincial ministry.

There is one notable exception to the seeming consensus in attendant service advocacy in Ontario: a small, radical group with little publicity or formal organization called DAMN (Disability Action Movement Now) 2025 (DAMN 2025 2008; Henderson 2007). Some of DAMN's efforts regarding Direct Funding are aimed at CILT. While still rejecting care, members of DAMN 2025 claim that the way CILT administers the program is "blatantly discriminatory against people who are illiterate. Many, many people with disabilities fit this description because of being segregated into institutions and 'special schools' where their abilities (both mental and physical) are underestimated and discouraged" (Ann Abbot, pers. comm.). The agendas of many other disability organizations include poverty, but DAMN consistently integrates a class analysis, keeping it at the forefront of radical disability politics and thus echoing the new wave of disability justice politics (Mingus 2011). The significance of DAMN's critiques is incongruous with documented disability movements in Ontario and the rest of Canada – that is, with histories that document a generally unified approach to Direct Funding.

There are parallel activities in Ontario led primarily by parent advocates regarding the Special Services at Home (SSAH) program, established in 1982, which was formerly available for children with any type of impairment and for adults with developmental disabilities. In 2012, adult funding was separated into the Passport program, designed for people with developmental disabilities who are eighteen years and older. SSAH is run through the Ontario Ministry of Children and Youth Services, whereas Passport funding is administered by the Ontario Ministry of Community and Social Services. Both programs provide funds to facilitate community participation, and the eligible expenses are much broader than those allowed by the Direct Funding Program. There is a long history of community-based advocacy aimed at the Ontario government, which includes asking for reduced waiting lists, increased funding, and, at one point, expanding eligibility of SSAH to children with physical disabilities (SSAH Provincial Coalition 2011). More recently, efforts have transitioned towards requests for a holistic individualized funding model to serve these constituencies (Individualized Funding Coalition for Ontario 2008) and for continuity between child and adult services. This does not suggest there is a unified approach to Direct Funding in Ontario, since the parent advocates do not push CILT or the Ministry of Health and Long Term Care to expand eligibility criteria for the Direct Funding program to include children or adults with intellectual disabilities. However, it does signify the popularity of direct and individualized funding options within disability spheres in Ontario, these options having a history that predates the pilot of Ontario's Direct Funding Program (SSAH Provincial Coalition 2011).

The Policy Landscape: From Neoliberalism to Austerity

In policy and in official state rhetoric, the Global North shifted to a neoliberal framework from the early 1990s onwards (Harvey 2005). In the most rudimentary sense, neoliberalism is a governing framework that privileges free markets and leads to the privatization of services. This results in smaller governments, at least rhetorically, since in practice neoliberal governance is characterized by increased surveillance of both citizens and noncitizens (Dobrowolsky 2008; Bhandar 2004; Stasiulis 2004). Ideologically, neoliberalism includes an emphasis on individual responsibility and exalts the value of choice for worker- and consumer-citizens (Mol 2006; Breitkreuz 2005; Larner 2000). Of relevance to disability movements with a long history in the nonprofit sector, neoliberal agendas are also linked to a co-optation of the third sector through a shift from core-funding arrangements to project-based competitions that are directly linked to government priorities (Incite! Women of Color against Violence 2007; M. Smith 2005; Hall and Banting 2000) and through the removal of gender from policy agendas (Brodie 2008). This period is also characterized by a transition away from full-time secure employment arrangements to more precarious forms of temporary, contractual, and part-time employment, which is reflected in the nature of attendant work under Direct Funding (Vosko 2000). Against the backdrop of these more localized trends is increased immigration and the exploitation of labour in the Global South to support the globalized economy (Encalada, Fuchs, and Paz 2008).

The neoliberal regime is accelerating and transforming in the wake of the 2008 global recession, which resulted in high unemployment that particularly affected young people in North America and Europe, and in damages to middle-class retirement savings, thus contributing to the aging workforce and delayed retirements. Government agendas refocused to bail out major industries, stimulate the economy, and implement austerity measures that would curb government spending by reducing social and health services. There were grassroots protests to these decisions, including the amorphous and largely misunderstood Occupy Wall Street movement that began in July 2011 and spread throughout the United States and into Canada over the summer and fall of that year (Chappell 2011).

In the United Kingdom and Greece, students filled the streets to protest specific austerity measures and demand access to education and employment. After the mass protest outside the Conservative Party conference on October 3, 2010, in Birmingham, England, the group Disabled People against Cuts, or DPAC, formed (2014). DPAC engages in a range of political tactics, from direct action to producing research and policy papers. DPAC has renewed disabled activism in the United Kingdom, and its work and popularity highlight how austerity policy frameworks disproportionately affect disabled people. Ellen Clifford(2014), a vocal leader within DPAC, reports that disabled people are nine times more likely to be directly affected by austerity measures than are nondisabled people, and that that number raises to nineteen times in relation to the most profoundly disabled and sick people. Further, Clifford emphasizes how cuts and dubiously applied policy changes result in the death, including by suicide, of disabled people. DPAC has mobilized a movement with over forty-five hundred formal members and a much broader base of support (Clifford 2014). DPAC garnered mainstream media attention during the 2012 Paralympic Games held in London by protesting the sponsorship involvement of Atos, a company contracted by the UK government to implement a harsh austerity measure, the Work Capability Assessment. This process claimed to determine whether people were fit for work and eligible for benefits, though DPAC discovered that the process was intended to reduce the overall provision of benefits and even included weekly quotas to ensure fewer people received support (Clifford 2014). Unfortunately, recommendations from the 2012 report by the Commission for the Review of Social Assistance in Ontario echo austerity trends in the United Kingdom, and it remains to be seen how these recommendations will play out in the Ontario context (Lankin and Sheikh 2012).[7] The ongoing visibility and presence of DPAC in the United Kingdom underscore the dire outcomes of austerity budgets for disabled and sick persons, and also the ability of disabled people to push back.

The shift to austerity has a varied effect on direct-funding schemes in the United Kingdom, which has an expansive Direct Payment program that is open to a wide variety of applicants, including older people, people with developmental disabilities, children with disabilities, people with mental health concerns, and adults with physical disabilities. The program, begun in 1997, expanded in 2003 when it became mandatory for all local councils to offer this option. Despite increases in enrolment in the early 2000s, interest in receiving

---

[7] For example, the report recommends that the province should "more vigorously pursue medical reviews of ODSP [Ontario Disability Support Program] recipients, and develop a strategy to deal with the backlog of reviews as a priority" (Lankin and Sheikh 2012, 103). If this strategy is taken up, the vigorous emphasis on medical reviews will perpetuate long-standing stereotypes about people with disabilities cheating the government support system and will likely result in ODSP recipients losing benefits in erratic and unfair ways, similar to what is happening in the United Kingdom.

Direct Payments remains lower than expected (Hall 2011). In addition to Direct Payments, a national Independent Living Fund (ILF) was set up by the Department of Social Security in 1988 to provide supplementary income with which people with disabilities could hire personal assistants. The ILF could be used in combination with Direct Payments or home care programs. Like Ontario's Direct Funding Program, the ILF and Direct Payments are tied to a history of Independent Living movements and activism, and the activist rationale for direct-payment schemes centred on cost-effectiveness, quality, and rights (Evans 2003).

In March 2014, the Tory-led coalition government announced the closure of the ILF, which at the time was funding approximately nineteen thousand disabled people. The government had previously attempted to close the fund in 2012 but was delayed after a protracted legal battle (Eady 2014). Disability activists are concerned this closure will mean less funding available to individual disabled people and result in more residential care options. The elimination of the ILF may signify an attempt to erase the connection to the Independent Living movement by removing the phrase "Independent Living" and by folding disabled people in with all other care recipients. In many ways, the cost-effectiveness and individualized focus of direct-funding schemes is a favourable policy option within an austerity framework, and yet simultaneously there is a deliberate erasure of the social movement history and social justice potential.

In this climate, direct-funding initiatives contribute to enduring neoliberal government priorities since they are extreme forms of downshifting service provision to individual citizens. Instead of provision of services by government-regulated and -owned institutions, care homes, or home care, money is transferred to the nonprofit sector (in the Ontario case), which administers the funds and, in turn, further shifts the services to individuals. It is the individual who becomes responsible for hiring and training other individuals to provide the personal support he or she requires. Disability movements in Ontario and elsewhere advocate strongly for the adoption of direct-funding mechanisms, thereby supporting the argument that social movements are agents in the enactment of neoliberal governmentality (Larner 2000). While direct-funding models of support may greatly benefit individuals with disabilities in a day-to-day sense, endorsing the neoliberal approach undermines other disability supports, changes the agendas of disability organizations, and contributes to the hostile environment for social movement activity.

Home care in Ontario and elsewhere in Canada has also been transformed by neoliberalism and austerity, through varied incremental processes that Hugh

Armstrong (2001) terms "privatization by stealth."[8] Aronson, Denton, and Zeytinoglu (2004) identify a "contractual approach" to home care in Ontario that promotes privatization linked to the landmark Commission on the Future of Health Care in Canada – colloquially known as the Romanow Commission (Health Canada 2009). Aronson and colleagues note that the commission made a "relatively weak and permissive recommendation[,] once again leaving supportive home care to the discretion of the provinces," and thus contributing to the privatized, contractual shift in home care and cementing the move to regionalization across all provinces (Aronson, Denton, and Zeytinoglu 2004, 113; see also Shapiro 2003; Jenson and Phillips 2000).

One development in health care reform in Ontario affecting attendant services is the 2005 adoption of the Local Health Integration Networks, or LHINs, following a similar approach in other provinces (Ronson 2006). There are fourteen LHINs in Ontario, delineated by geography, whose primary activity is to streamline health care services by making funding decisions for various health-related organizations (Ronson 2006). The ministry moved "from a system manager to a system planning and oversight role" (Ronson 2006, 47) – another example of the changing role of governments in the neoliberal context. This is a system-wide shift in health care administration; yet, despite being funded by the same ministry, until 2011, the Direct Funding Program managed to bypass this mechanism because of its provincial scope – one of its most lauded features – as well as because of the relatively small number of people it serves. The program is now under the LHINs system, but incorporating it required a change to accommodate programs with a provincial scope. Furthermore, during this shift, CILT confirmed program materials (which reject "care") and maintained control over the administration of the funds. The Direct Funding Program clearly fits within broader trends of neoliberalism and austerity, yet it uniquely manages to maintain a semblance of autonomy and philosophical commitments to Independent Living, unlike developments in the United Kingdom.

From this brief review, it is clear that local to global policy landscapes are constantly changing, with frequent adjustments to political positions, policy

---

[8] In principle, CILT seeks to distance Ontario's Direct Funding Program from other forms of home care and long-term care, instead presenting the idea of attendant services. In practice, the distance may not be so great; many self-managers previously used other services and, in the case of home care, some access it simultaneously or intermittently while receiving direct funding. Furthermore, the Ministry of Health and Long-Term Care funds the entire system and categorizes Direct Funding as a form of long-term care.

responses, and budgetary priorities, regardless of which government is elected to power or which international body is in discussion. Disabled people, like other marginalized and abject populations, are approached as a special-interest group to be catered to, consulted with in prescribed formats, or ignored, depending on the potential votes or perceived political ramifications of these actions. On a provincial level, attendant services and other forms of support become one more budget line and policy-briefing topic to be considered and continually deferred, while the experiences of the services are often inadequate, especially for those on waiting lists. Political attention and seeming gains, such as the 2014 injection of capital into the Direct Funding Program or the budgetary announcement of a wage increase for personal support workers (Sousa 2014), follow prolonged periods where people are in crisis, waiting on wait lists, or dealing with high worker turnover because of low wages.[9] Titchkosky (2011, 93) comments: "An abiding concern is how, under bureaucratic governance including legislative or procedural change, disability remains more or less represented as an unexpected participant." The presence of disabled people and discussions of social supports for people with disabilities in political arenas is not only unexpected but often optional for politicians. In this context, Titchkosky makes a compelling argument that "disability is managed as a potentially excludable phenomenon since it is present as a not-yet" (109). In the "not yet" time of disability, bodily difference is submerged into a liberal (and timeless) notion of a universal public body while, at the same time, the specifics of disability are never important or present enough to be a pressing political priority. Titchkosky argues that this erasure happens even in bureaucratic responses that are specifically about disability, such as the Accessibility for Ontarians with Disabilities Act (AODA), which notably does not promise an accessible Ontario "now" but twenty years from its establishment, in 2025. The policies, consultations, and detailed measurements legislated into law attempt to usher in social inclusion and publicly signify "action" by political leaders, while disabled people remain literally absent from positions of power and even from mundane (but meaningful) activities of daily life. As governments change and budgets are announced, minor adjustments may be made to policies and programs that

---

9 The wage increase initially excluded attendants working under Direct Funding, Special Services at Home, and Passport. Setting attendant services apart from other forms of care has the potential to be a politically and culturally salient strategy, yet it can also have material consequences when direct-funding options are excluded from broader policy developments.

dramatically shape the lives of disabled people, but disability and care remains "not yet" a priority.

Shifts in Social Policy and Medicine

There are parallel moves among governments to adopt direct-funding options or to use voucher systems instead of providing services in social policy and health spheres. Voucher systems have been implemented in childcare systems (e.g., Warner and Gradus 2011; Adams, Rohacek, and Snyder 2008) and education (e.g., Witte 2000; King, Orazem, and Wohlgemuth 1999). For example, Martin Carnoy (1998, 335) finds mixed results from education vouchers, arguing they do not achieve what the supporters claim but also do not signify the "catastrophic decline in public education claimed by its opponents." Carnoy further notes that the national voucher systems he explores are tied to political agendas and linked to an overall decrease in educational contributions from governments, which also resonates with the low-cost argument linked to direct-funding programs for people with disabilities.

Another important related development is the increasing emphasis on "patient-centred," "patient-directed," "person-centred," "client-centred," or "consumer-directed" care in medical fields and in some educational approaches to disability (e.g., Macleod and McPherson 2007; Turner-Stokes 2007; Davis et al. 2005; Nolin and Killackey 2004). Although difficult to define precisely, patient-centred care includes an implicit critique of the power and control given to medical professionals through the current organization of medical systems. Patient-centred care attempts to level power imbalances by providing information to enable patients to make their own health care decisions (with the added incentive for medical practitioners to pass on the liability for those decisions). Evidence shows that patient-centred approaches lead to more satisfactory experiences with medical systems and, theoretically, to better care (Sidani 2008).

Patient-centred care requires a change in values and assumptions, and conflicts with the more dominant trend of evidence-based medicine (Bensing 2000). According to Lewis (2009), the shift requires understanding patients as a type of consumer, and health care as the provision of services. This resonates with the ideas behind the concept of attendant services. Despite the emphasis on the "good of the patient," patient-centred approaches also intend to decrease physician and practitioner liability, decrease health care costs, and in some respects, maintain an aura of paternalism, as the professionals must counsel and encourage self-determination and self-care among the patients, who are presumed to lack these skills.

Patient-centred medical approaches may not be as popular as evidence-based ones, particularly in practice, and may have more complex intentions than first appear; nevertheless, it is a notable trend that demonstrates a hospitable climate for direct-funding models of attendant services. The emphasis on decision making and patient knowledge, and the occasional drift into market-based consumer terminology, make direct-funding options appear to be a patient-centred approach to long-term home care. Patient-centred care emphasizes individual needs and specific localized contexts; however, care policies and work are also valuable commodities in a globalized world.

Globalization and Care

Care work is globalized in ways that include the physical migration of workers to care-related fields and, more conceptually, the exchange of social and health policy frameworks across borders and political contexts. The latter can be seen in multinational, comparative academic studies of direct funding (e.g., Adams, Rohacek, and Snyder 2008; Ungerson and Yeandle 2007; Carnoy 1998), and it would be inaccurate to claim that Ontario's Direct Funding Program emerged without reference to these other contexts. Since the majority of migrants are now women entering gendered forms of work, the trend of migrating workers is of great interest to feminist researchers (Parreñas 2008; Zimmerman, Litt, and Bose 2006). The migration of women to perform service and care work often signifies an inequality among the women in receiving countries, the migrant women, and, even more pronounced, the women who stay behind to perform care duties in the home countries. The demand for care workers in receiving countries "also speaks of women's oppressions in neoliberal states and the failure of states to meet the needs of women who choose to enter the labor force" (Parreñas 2008, 137).

In Canada, which is considered a receiving country, there is a federal initiative known as the Live-in Caregiver Program designed to attract foreign domestic workers to support children, older people, and sometimes people with physical disabilities (Tumolva and Tomeldan 2004; Stasiulis and Bakan 1997; Bakan and Stasiulis 1994). The Direct Funding Program operates independently of this program, and the number of temporary or new Canadians employed through Direct Funding is not well documented. The only available demographic information on attendants is from the 1997 evaluation of the Direct Funding pilot. The 1995–96 pilot version of the program served 102 self-managers from across Ontario and documents 16 percent of self-managers' main attendants as being visible minorities, and 10 percent as being people who did not speak French of English as a first language (with a likely overlap in those percentages); it does not provide information on country of birth (Roeher Institute 1997). Further, the financial administrative start-up package published by CILT allows for the hiring of people with temporary work permits (CILT 2008, 4). Ontario's Direct Funding Program has globalized connections conceptually and more concretely through the individual histories of the attendants, though this remains an important area for further inquiry.

Among these various trends – the developments in disability movements in Canada and elsewhere; the influence of neoliberalism, austerity, and health care reform; shifts towards voucher and direct-funding services and patient-centred care; and the globalization of care policy and work – the Direct Funding Program in many ways fits in. It might at first appear unremarkable that disability advocates in Ontario were able to secure and maintain funding for this program. However, what is remarkable is that community advocates and an organization with a social movement history were able to set the terms and continue to maintain a significant degree of control over the program. Material on the Direct Funding Program includes strong cultural messages about disability, care, and empowerment that might not otherwise appear if the program were administered in a more distanced, "objective" fashion by a government ministry or even by a nonprofit organization with a less political history. There will be an opportunity to explore parallel examples that do not have this history in the coming years as the Ontario government pilots programs for seniors. The Direct Funding Program does not represent a concession or a straight-forward manifestation of neoliberal ideologies, which often serve to dismantle social movements (M. Smith 2005). Rather, the program helps set the agenda for, and stands out as a unique example among, broad trends that can seem unruly at times.

Organization of *Disability Politics and Care*

Throughout this book, I make the case that the rejection of care in public rhetoric related to Ontario's Direct Funding Program, and in other similar programs and advocacy efforts worldwide, is only part of the story. The rejection of care does not eliminate it but moves it to appropriate realms, thus limiting its oppressive and invasive potentials. It may be disconcerting to some to define "care" as *also* a form of oppression, but this book aims to thoroughly engage with the critique raised by people with disabilities and disability scholars, and explore what it might mean to incorporate this critique into discussions and practices of care.

Part 1 provides theoretical and methodological tools for understanding care and direct funding. Chapter 1 uses elements of autoethnography to theorize an informal support relationship between me and "Killian," a friend with a physical disability who uses direct funding. Given my experience in our particular "frientendant" relationship, I argue that the common scholarly orientations towards care do not adequately explain our situation. Starting from the conversations between feminist and disability perspectives on care, I develop the theoretical framework of *accessible care*. Accessible care takes a critical, engaged approach that moves beyond understanding accessibility as merely concrete solutions, to create more inclusive forms of care. Care, in this context, is positioned as an unstable tension among competing definitions, including that it is a complex form of oppression. Accessible care draws on feminist disability perspectives and feminist political ethics of care to build bridges in four areas: from daily experiences of disability and support to theoretical discussions; across feminist care research and disability perspectives; across divisions and anxieties within disability communities; and from the local to transnational applications. These bridges do not aim to resolve debates but allow us to travel back and forth between differing perspectives and demonstrate the tenuous possibility of accessible practices and conceptualizations of care.

Chapter 2 considers qualitative research as a form of care, one that requires us to be constantly aware of the potential to slide towards coercion. The specific examples from this study can also inform a broader discussion about research dynamics. I argue that the interpersonal dilemmas faced in qualitative research are not isolated occurrences but are reflective of a powerful research industry that includes a history of oppression and ongoing social inequalities.

Part 2 addresses the initial aim of this study, that is, to sketch contemporary forms of care by exploring Ontario's Direct Funding Program. Generally, this study finds that care is not what happens "here" within the program or within attendant services more broadly. Distinct concepts are used to describe the interactions between disabled people and their attendants. However, the subsequent chapter reveals the "authentic times to care," the meanings and practices that remain classified as care amid this passionate rejection.

Chapter 3 focuses on what care is *not*, based on the interview and contextual material. I first present the material demonstrating that attendant services are not care, as care encompasses too much and not enough to describe what is happening under Direct Funding. I then sketch aspects of the daily interactions between attendants and self-managers in order to create a reference for "non-care."

The attendants fulfill multiple roles in the lives of the self-managers and their work is described both as concrete "arms and legs" activities and in relational terms. The concrete tasks of attendant services are done under the direction of the self-manager, thereby easing the attendants' sense of responsibility during interactions, while relational ties simultaneously raise attendants' sense of responsibility off-hours to ensure they do not miss shifts. The relational aspects are a mandatory part of attendant work and are distinguished from notions of care, despite emotional and empathetic descriptors. Specific examples of interpersonal techniques deployed by self-managers and attendants show that relational ontologies are formed within attendant services.

Even though the majority of participants in this study reject the term "care" in some way, Chapter 4 argues that this rejection does not mean that care completely disappears. Very few of the participants avoid the term entirely, and some imply that there are places where care belongs. Care emerges as an ambiguous set of actions and attitudes that we all have to tolerate at some points in our lives. I explore four key areas that still count as care. (1) Care is an intricate form of oppression; (2) it is linked to medical and social professionals; (3) it is a necessary set of actions during times of illness, for specialized medical treatments, and for highly intimate needs; and finally, (4) it is an approach to supporting people with intellectual disabilities and others who cannot self-direct.

The meanings of care are refined and contained in the Direct Funding Program, and doing so challenges theoretical debates among feminist and disability scholars. The findings challenge the polemic of independence/attendant services and interdependence/care by demonstrating that there are still places in which care belongs. Removing care from Independent Living attendant services does not erase it, but changes the meanings and practices associated with it.

Part 3 turns to the tangible implications of the removal of care. Although the theoretical contributions to care scholarship matter in the realm of cultural meaning making, there are also more concrete consequences of this process in the broader policy landscape. Chapter 5 highlights the policy connections related to the removal of care. The chapter argues that removing care can obfuscate the limitations of the program, the basic provision of disability supports, and transnational issues. Yet the critiques of care from Independent Living have a unique potential to intervene in other policy topics by bringing forth rights-based and alternative perspectives on health. For example, there is a distancing and even rejection of professionalization for Direct Funding attendants, but a respect for the necessary role of health professionals in the lives of the self-managers. This creates an intricate and at times ambiguous relationship to professionals that is not often acknowledged in provincial conversations about education and regulation of Personal Support Workers. Efforts to critique and reject care may not always be considered in policy discussions, but they the hold the potential to (and sometimes do) challenge and intervene with critically embodied and politicized insights.

Chapter 6 explores the implications of a nonprofit organization affiliated with the Independent Living movement administering a government-funded program. The cultural critiques of care and other aspects of the Independent Living movement do not evolve in administrative documents, which are accountable to ministry oversight. As such, the removal of care from attendant services diverges from evolving approaches to disability policy, as well as from a new generation of activists. Although, practically, Direct Funding fits among a number of policy trends, as identified earlier, it appears incongruous with recent developments in the disability sector, such as the Ontario-based transformation of developmental services, and the motivations behind the UN Convention on the Rights of Persons with Disabilities. Outside the policy realm, the rejection of care and the administrative role of Independent Living does not align with the approaches of an emerging generation of disability activists engaging in disability justice work (Mingus 2011). I detail a parallel project, the Youth Activist Forum, to demonstrate that new leaders exist but that the Independent Living model does not always make room for the issues and approaches they represent.

To conclude the book, I explore removing care amid a "care crisis" for older people that dominates popular and policy discourses. Directly-funded home care is often cited as a potential solution to this crisis, yet it further entrenches neoliberal frameworks and worldviews, complete with other crises of austerity. The Direct Funding Program changes the experiences of support in Ontario and challenges common understandings of care. And yet, the program cannot be interpreted as a simple success story, as it has notable limitations, including creating highly precarious forms of labour for the attendants. The removal of care and endorsement of direct-funding policy approaches does not resolve all oppressive practices of care and the adamant distancing from care may not resonate with evolving disability movements in Canada and elsewhere.

PART 1

Conceptualizing and Researching Care

1

Accessible Care

Killian is a good friend, a man with a physical disability, and a self-manager under the Direct Funding Program.[1] I identify as a woman, and strive to be a nondisabled ally. Awkwardly but naturally, it came to pass that I occasionally help him eat or use the washroom. This is mostly done informally, as a friend, but on one or two occasions, Killian paid me to assist him. Even when the arrangement is more formal, Killian articulates that he is uncomfortable calling me his attendant and insists "friend" is more appropriate. We joke that "frientendant" is perhaps the most accurate term. Outside of our relationship, I am intrigued by the process whereby Killian's attendants (sometimes) become his friends, his friends become attendants, or people around him increasingly lend a hand in tasks not normally associated with friendship.

Although I had previous interest in and experiences with disability, considering Killian and his relationships with his attendants influenced my interpretation of scholarship on Independent Living, home care, social policy, and care as an ethical and theoretical concept. I found that our specific relationship did not quite fit into most of these accounts. This is not to claim that our in/formal interactions are the standard, but rather to reveal cracks in existing literature and use it as an entry point to discuss broader issues relating to independence and care. I do not claim to speak for Killian; my account of our relationship is partial, with details escaping or becoming idealized on the page. Partiality from an allied position, however, does not mean irrelevance (L. Davis 1995).

[1] "Killian" is a pseudonym.

The snapshots I provide of varied disability and feminist perspectives on care, along with a more detailed account of the conversations between the two, highlight how they speak to (or do not speak to) my and Killian's relationship. Inspired by concepts in feminist disability studies and the feminist political ethics of care, I argue that we must make care *accessible*. In previous work, I suggest accessible care "builds bridges, which are not necessarily intended to dwell on points of agreement" (Kelly 2011, 564); in this chapter, I further develop this concept and outline the four areas these bridges span:

1. From daily experiences of disability and care to theoretical discussions
2. Across feminist care research and disability perspectives
3. Across divisions and anxieties within disability communities
4. From the local to the transnational context.

By building bridges in these areas, accessible care advances the theoretical idea, policy implications, and practices of care in ways that engage with disability perspectives without abandoning the work of feminist care researchers. Most substantially, accessible care frames scholarly discussions of attendant services for people with disabilities more sufficiently than an exclusive Independent Living, feminist ethics, or other feminist care orientation. Further, accessible care can serve to challenge and stimulate studies and discussions of the many forms of care (e.g., policy, practice, theory) for other groups of people and types of workers.

Perspectives on Care

The first time I helped Killian eat, I knew we were no longer simply friends, and it was at times awkward for us to negotiate our shifting roles as we became increasingly entangled in the gendered politics of care. We were at a national-level adaptive sports tournament. My partner is also a person with a physical disability and at the time played competitive sports, which is how we met Killian. My partner does not need much assistance at meals or during games, which allowed me to assist Killian and other athletes at the multiday event. On the final evening, the organizers hosted a banquet and gave out the medals and awards. Killian's paid attendant, also a friend of his in this case, was noticeably tired from assisting Killian during the games and supporting him with other daily tasks. I asked Killian if I instead could help him eat, and I nervously fumbled to figure out an appropriate rhythm of cutting food, asking what he wanted next and when he was ready for it, and delivering bites from plate to mouth while trying to eat my own meal too. I had helped many others eat before, but I found it difficult to interact with a relatively new friend in such an intimate way. Killian smiled and bantered throughout the meal, and he expertly demonstrated his skill at putting new able-bodied frien-tendants at ease.

How can we understand what was happening between Killian and me? Divergent scholarship related to care reveals substantive epistemic tensions, especially among disability scholars and feminists. Independent Living perspectives distance personal assistance from caring for children, sick people, and older people, and highlight the empowering nature of consumer-directed models of support (e.g., Stainton and Boyce 2004; Beatty et al. 1998; Zarb and Nadash 1994). Independent Living ultimately aims to shift control of services to those who require them and promotes an employer-employee relationship. This material offers valuable concepts relevant to me and Killian, particularly because he uses an Independent Living model of support and his specific arrangement is partly, or largely, the result of the efforts of local and international disability activists (Yoshida et al. 2004). Their demands and achievements echo throughout our interactions, as I am ever aware of the importance for Killian to be the one in charge. Yet, this model has limits. When I helped him at the banquet, we were not interacting on a purely employer-employee basis, he was not directing every action that took place, and our relationship and interactions encompassed more than independence.

Related theoretical work in disability studies implicitly and explicitly positions care as a layered form of oppression that includes abuse, coercion, a history of physical and metaphorical institutionalization, and a denial of agency often signified by excluding disabled people from research (e.g., Longmore 2003; Linton 1998; L. Davis 1995; Oliver 1983). Although it seems appropriate in Killian's situation and for others using attendant services (e.g., Erickson 2007), the boundary crossings of the frien-tendant can also lead to difficult emotional disappointments and misunderstandings. Indeed, as disability scholarship so effectively demonstrates, the potential for daily practices of care to veer into pain and oppression is high. Awareness of this history and potential explains many aspects of our relationship, such as why Killian hires by word of mouth and why it is so important for him to direct his personal support. But the disability critiques of care also have limits, as they often ignore the gendered nature of care work and the potential coercion and abuse of the individuals who work as care providers, many of whom are transnational and racialized subjects.

Largely unconnected to disability studies, numerous feminist empirical studies position care as a gendered form of work that needs to be revalued. These studies document the experiences of different types of formal and informal care workers, conduct policy analyses of care delivery systems, and typically focus on the perspectives of the workers (e.g., Tumolva and Tomeldan 2004; Macdonald and Merrill 2002; Stasiulis and Bakan 1997). More recently, feminist care scholars highlight the transnational nature of contemporary forms of care work (e.g., Zimmerman, Litt, and Bose 2006). Feminist scholarship on care work is sometimes difficult to apply to the relationship between Killian and me, as it largely focuses on the perspectives of those who provide support; in practice, as a self-manager, Killian plays an integral administrative role in the services. The tendency to underemphasize the agency of the recipient of support in care dynamics is the central critique levelled at feminists by disability scholars.

Finally, a (sometimes) related body of literature attempts to theorize care broadly (e.g., Duffy 2005; Daly 2002). More specifically, there is a contested ethics of care perspective that positions care as a moral framework grounded in the daily experiences of providing care, most often to children. Gilligan (1982) and Noddings (1984) are most consistently cited as laying the foundations of this perspective. Gilligan observes that the field of psychology was seemingly premised on men's experiences of the world. In particular, as girls were (eventually) included in Kohlberg's studies of childhood moral development (1981), their responses to the moral dilemmas typically scored at level three out of six on a progressive trajectory. Gilligan argued that it was not the moral capacities of the female participants that were flawed but Kohlberg's model. Gilligan's ethics of care emerged as a relational, concrete, and active set of decision-making tools, as opposed to the abstract, rule-based ethics of justice that dominates the field of moral philosophy as well as common systems of morality. Relationships between these two ethics would later become the subject for many of the debates in this area (e.g., Clement 1996; Kroeger-Mappes 1994; Manning 1992).

Noddings's version of care ethics (1984) argues that we have an obligation to care, and that that obligation is greater for those with whom we are already in a relationship or with whom there is a potential future relationship. Noddings strongly resists the idea of abstract ethical rules, arguing that moral decisions must be made in context, and thus contributes to the development of a flexible and difficult-to-teach "rationality of caring" (Waerness 1996). There is a specific focus on the daily, relational elements of care and a rejection of care as a political concept, as is made clear when Noddings (1984, 103) declares that "no institution or nation can be ethical."

The foundation of this literature did not stand for long; many critiques surfaced, particularly stemming from Noddings's early work. For example, in an oft-cited article resonating with disability critiques of care, Card (1990) argues that Noddings's approach risks valorizing abusive relationships, since care is placed as a moral imperative above all else, making it difficult to end any type of relationship. A further critique of Noddings comes from Manning (1992, 72): "The claim that one must withdraw from the public sphere and retreat to the private when neglecting those to whom one is already related strikes me as [a] classic defence of the stereotypical role of the housewife." In more recent work, Noddings (2006) responds to critics by exploring care as a social policy tool. She suggests that we examine life in "ideal homes" as a starting point. She continues her critique of principles, though in contradiction offers several strong recommendations and universals, including advocating for the termination of potentially disabled fetuses.

Early ethics of care literature did not fully engage with the idea that care is a relationship. Many of the examples are written from the perspective of the "one-caring," to use Noddings's term, and easily assign the power to this person as the moral decision maker; if possible, the "cared for" is encouraged to amicably receive the actions of the "one-caring" to make her job more palatable. The issue is not just the framing of care as between two unequal parties but a historical and evolving body of scholarship that continually emphasizes the provision of care at the expense of the perspectives of those who require ongoing assistance with the tasks of daily living. It is these examples that seem the furthest from my experiences with Killian and consumer-directed models proposed by Independent Living movements. As the findings of this study show, some attendants do not want to be moral decision makers and enjoy the freedom from liability associated with following directions.

The ethics of care literature has further evolved in two main directions, one towards what Williams (2001) terms a feminist political ethics of care that pulls care away from everyday moral decision making to a political framework; the other, towards work on dependency. Political ethics of care work responds to many critiques of early ethics of care scholarship, expanding our understandings of care beyond two-party relationships. For example, Marion Barnes (2006, 178) writes that it is not "empirically accurate nor morally defensible to define people as only givers or receivers of care." Instead, the feminist political ethics of care asserts that care should become a central civic value (Tronto 2013, 1993; Mahon and Robinson 2011; Engster 2007; Lawson 2007; Robinson 2006, 1999; Held 2005; Harrington 2000; Sevenhuijsen 1998;). The implications of endorsing such a position are ripe with potential benefits for disabled people and are explored later in this chapter.

Another development in ethics of care literature is work on dependency, led by Eva Feder Kittay, a feminist philosopher who draws on her experiences as a mother of a daughter with profound intellectual and physical disabilities. For Kittay (1999), care is an inherently unequal relationship that maintains the "foundational myths," as Fineman (2004) puts it, of contemporary society by masking the inevitable dependencies of life. Kittay uses the term "dependent" to refer to those who require assistance and suggests that dependents are "the charge" of care workers, which leaves little room for any expression of agency on behalf of those receiving help. This may apply to some disabled people who communicate in nonverbal ways or require assistance to make decisions, but it does not account for people who need daily assistance and are able to make decisions about their lives. It certainly does not apply to Killian. It would be simply offensive and demeaning to refer to Killian as "my charge." Nonetheless, Kittay's contribution helps demonstrate the degrees and varieties of dependence, independence, and interdependence by centring people, like her daughter, who are so often excluded from other frameworks.

Scholarship related to "care" and the many other applications of the term are extensive and far surpass what I have pointed to here. When approached as discrete bodies of literature, each scholarly grouping leaves many aspects of the relationship between Killian and me under- or unexplained; however, a fifth, small body of work can be considered as conversations among the above groupings. This chapter advances these conversations, which are at times hostile, more recently sympathetic, and the starting point for forging accessible versions of care.

Conversations

The few conversations among the bodies of work signify other Killians, that is, voices that demonstrate the limitations of the common scholarly approaches to care work, theory, and ethics.

The earliest and ongoing conversations between feminists and disability scholars (often also feminists) are characterized by silence on the part of the former, or hostility on both parts. Disability scholars or, arguably, feminist disability scholars, first critiqued researchers and theorists working in the field of care not only for ignoring the perspective of people with disabilities but also for further disabling people through oppressive representations in their work (e.g., Morris 2001; Silvers 1997). Thomas (2007) recounts several confrontations that took place at academic conferences in the United Kingdom, including the dismissal by some scholars of disability perspectives as minority viewpoints that were not practical or important. After witnessing such overt hostility,

Thomas (2007, 119) concludes: "The disciplinary divide remains wide and deep on questions of care and dependency: the social oppression and social deviance paradigms clash irreconcilably."

In light of this history, I try to be cautious with my use of autoethnography, to avoid replicating the limitations of care scholarship written from or about the perspective of the workers. I asked permission from Killian before writing about him but continue to struggle with how to represent him fairly, as I explore in the subsequent chapter.

In other conversations, scholars engage with both disability and feminist perspectives, but they implicitly or explicitly conclude that feminist approaches to care work are the most adequate (Beckett 2007; M. Barnes 2006). A few scholars writing from a cultural theory perspective also end up abandoning Independent Living perspectives on care (e.g., Fritsch 2010; Gibson 2006; Price and Shildrick 2002). This work is promising in that it acknowledges that disability critiques of care exist, but it still ends up dismissing this perspective, sometimes more thoroughly than others. Conversations where disability scholarship and organizations "lose" in an academic forum do not seem to fully acknowledge the efforts and cultural messages of disability activists who argue "We do not need care."

The final theme is more recent, with Wendell (1996) representing an early example. In this conversation, scholars engage with both disability and feminist perspectives and attempt to salvage and protect each viewpoint in order to build bridges and lay the foundations for new approaches (Kröger 2009; Shakespeare 2006; Hughes et al. 2005; Watson et al. 2004; Garland-Thomson 2002, 16–17; Williams 2001), and this perspective is trickling into empirical studies (Gibson et al. 2009). This work affirms the relationship between Killian and me by highlighting that "disabled people and their assistants do not experience personal assistance in purely contractual, unemotional and instrumental terms" (Watson et al. 2004, 338). This small detail is a significant opportunity for bridging the independence-interdependence divide, similar to feminist work on relational autonomy (e.g., Clement 1996). That this conversation draws on the "feminist voice in disability studies" indicates that disability scholarship includes more than just Independent Living (Hughes et al. 2005, 259) and makes room for both/and instead of either/or (Shakespeare 2006). Indeed, in light of these developments and in contrast to Thomas's assessment (2007), Kröger (2009, 406) asserts: "The fundamental conceptual antagonism between care research and disability studies seems to have become diluted recently." At the point where the tension is diluted and the scholars actively engage with one another, we can begin to build accessible care.

Accessible Care

If approached cautiously, accessibility can be a powerful concept; it has been mobilized and transformed by disability activists, becoming a central concept in disability-related policy and legislation and a signpost for spaces that take disability seriously. Most often, "accessibility" refers to adapting physical and social environments to be more inclusive of disabled people. When done properly, accessibility is not mere logistics, despite highly specific standards outlined in accessibility legislation. The risk of accessibility, however, is that it may inadvertently focus on people with physical disabilities, or transform disability into a fixable problem rather than a complex cultural category.

Titchkosky (2011, 3) explores the question of access in the university setting. She argues that access is not merely "a substance to be measured for its presence or absence" but is an "interpretative relation between bodies." It is thus possible for activist and legal work on accessibility to bridge into theoretical work on the nature of disability and inclusion. The most radical, critical forms of accessibility must be handled *with care* – that is, with a vigilant defence against valuable, inclusive social justice concepts (e.g., accessibility) becoming diluted, co-opted, or process-oriented. Accessibility is not inherently linked to disability studies or even to disability movements; it can easily fall away from critical reflection into bureaucratic checklists addressing "complaints" or challenging design puzzles for engineers and other professionals linked primarily to physical impairments. "Careful," vigilantly critical approaches to access and accessibility, then, can help us explore the constant evolution of the meanings of varied embodiments. This careful approach to accessibility enables tangible environmental changes *and* facilitates critical reflection on how environments mirror underlying, often unquestioned social assumptions about disability. But accessibility, like care, is not enough to describe the relationship between people with disabilities and those who support them.

Care, as we have briefly explored, is a highly contested concept that is difficult to define. Fine (2007, 4) pushes against "singular definitions" of care and sets forth a complex definition that concludes: "In viewing care, however, what might be thought of as the negative or dark side of care, the enforced dependency of care-givers and the potential for harm to the recipient need to be recognized alongside the more positive attributes." Care cannot be reduced to a simple definition and, most significantly, the abusive side of care cannot be removed from academic and public understandings. Further, as the disability critiques of care reveal, the potential for oppressive care is much deeper than alluded to in Fine's definition, as it extends beyond daily abuse to firmly rooted institutionalized approaches to disability. Care scholars do address issues of violence *in relation* to care, but not as *a part* of it. For example, when writing about gendered aspects of masculine care, Joan Tronto (2013) implores, "How, especially if I am right that [care and violence] are at opposite ends of a spectrum of how humans should treat one another, can violence and care cohabit intimate space?" Although different from common understandings of care, this is not such an impossible question if the perspectives of disability scholars and activists are taken seriously. Indeed, care and help are intricately interwoven with violence, oppression, and harm. I am not suggesting this is the way it should be, but we must acknowledge the realities of care in order to avoid obfuscating oppressive experiences of care and to enable new visions of the future.

Feminist scholars also discuss the linkages between care and coercion, but unlike Fine's focus on interpersonal interactions and disability scholars' attention to the legacies of institutionalization, they emphasize how care work systematically disadvantages women. Evelyn Nakano Glenn (2010, 5), in particular, summarizes the key argument of her book:

> The social organization of care has been rooted in diverse forms of coercion that have induced women to assume responsibility for caring for family members and that have tracked poor, racial minority, and immigrant women into positions entailing caring for others. The forms of coercion have varied in degree, directness, and explicitness but nonetheless have served to constrain and direct women's choices; the net consequence of restricted choice has been to keep caring labour "cheap," that is, free (in the case of family care labour) or low waged (in the case of paid care labour).

Glenn's analysis connects the social organization of care within dominating systems of oppression in a contextualized socioeconomic framework. Glenn briefly engages with the disability movement (though not with the critiques of care) and notes that the movement sets "a precedent for claiming the right to *receive* care as essential for meaningful citizenship. What is more difficult is to make the case for rights and entitlements for those *providing* care" (Glenn 2010, 193). Care can be an abusive interaction between individuals rooted in specific situated power dynamics, an institutionalized approach to disability, *and* an unjust social organization that systematically disadvantages and devalues women by coercing us to provide formal and informal care. In all these ways, and many other specific examples, care can be dangerous, oppressive, and coercive; however, the provision of care also is an avenue to mediate meaningful participation in life, can create complex relationships, and can be a rewarding career path, among other positive intonations.

Building on Fine and Glenn, I suggest that care, specifically *accessible* care, is an unstable tension among emotions, actions, and values, simultaneously pulled towards both empowerment and coercion (see also Kelly 2011). "Coercion" in this context refers both to coercion and abuse among individuals, and to overarching systems of oppression such as the social organization of care work described by Glenn and the institutionalization and medicalization of disability. Care is a paradox (Douglas 2010a); it represents the failure of medical cure and neoliberal progress; it is a deep compassion and empathy, a highly intimate relationship, an institutionalized approach to disability, a transnational supply and demand of feminized labour, a dependency on state-funded programs, and so on. It is a tension among all these definitions, none to be disregarded. To distinguish this definition of care from our common usages requires the critical concept of access that reveals the links among discourse, material environments, and social inequalities. Accessibility, like care, is never fully achieved but requires continual evaluation of our practices and shared discourses on disability. Pairing (critical) accessibility with competing definitions positions care as a moving tension that cannot be resolved. Accessible care introduces a new approach to, and new applications of, care. This seemingly unwieldy definition captures the complexity of care, and significantly advances the conversations about care among feminist and disability scholars in ways that are particularly useful for discussing attendant services.

Building Bridges

Drawing on material from feminist disability studies and the feminist political ethics of care, I argue that accessible care builds bridges in four arenas. It works to account for daily experiences of disability and support provision in theoretical discussions; challenge feminist researchers to account for disability critiques while also encouraging disability scholars to consider feminist insights on care, thus positioning care as a tension; address exclusions and strains within disability studies and communities; and finally, position discussions of attendant services, and care, within transnational contexts. It is here that I return to Killian, as this formulation of care more adequately accounts for our relationship, among other applications.

Bridge One: From Daily Experiences to Theory

Accessible care is grounded in the daily, intersectional experiences of support provision, which can be used to formulate and evaluate theoretical discussions. This bridge resonates with feminist disability theorists who hold disability as an experiential social identity and a cultural category (Garland-Thomson 2002). Disability is both a lens through which to examine cultural artifacts and social phenomena, and a specific embodiment and minority identity. Significantly, many feminist definitions of disability build on social model and Independent Living perspectives rather than dismantle them or the tremendous material improvements achieved under those frameworks. As such, disability critiques of care emerging from an Independent Living perspective are still useful and serve as a valuable critique of care industries, medical institutions, and patronizing charitable approaches.

When exploring the experiential side of disability, feminist disability theorists highlight the value of embodied, personal accounts that emphasize the agency of people with disabilities. Although some people cannot provide first-hand narratives in written or oral formats, as is further discussed regarding bridge three, consumer control and making room for personal accounts of care honour the agency of those who can. Personal accounts also reveal the intersectional nature of support interactions (Clare 1999; Wendell 1996) and, more recently, the material-semiotic nature of these interactions (Garland-Thomson 2011; Schriempf 2001).[2] This complex intersectionality is essential for understanding the experiences of personal assistance, experiences that are visceral while also fraught with social meanings about gender, the body, race, class, sexuality, and ability.

Killian and I occupy similar social locations in terms of age, economic status, education, sexuality, and perceived race. Although our example may not be one of the rich locations for studying difference, as identified by Hillyer (1993), the intersections we do embody pervade our interactions. Even the third or fourth time I assisted Killian in the washroom, it was preceded by an uncomfortable debate about whether it was going to be weird for us, and I must admit that, in some ways, it *can* be weird for me. Inside the cramped public-bathroom stall, my social discomfort was palpable as I grasped for body language and

---

2 "Material-semiotic" refers to Schriempf's "interactionist" paradigm (2001) to understanding disability and impairment and follows Donna Haraway, arguing that "everything is 'always already' social and material" (68).

conversation appropriate within this context. Our debate and my experiences expose a common space within personal assistance where privacy, sexuality, and gender overlap and require delicate interpersonal negotiation that seems to require more skill and effort from Killian than from me as the frien-tendant (Marfisi 2010). These moments are awkward because they make us acutely aware of the layered power dynamics inherent in our female/male, disabled/nondisabled, and clothed/unclothed embodiments that we more typically prefer to ignore, since it brings the abusive potential of care uncomfortably close to the surface. As an individual who appears and identifies as a woman, I invoke the cultural figure of the female caregiver that I simultaneously embody and resist through my actions. Like disability, the actions of attendant work are not merely performative, as certain gestures must be completed in order to adequately meet Killian's needs. Whereas, for example, fork-to-mouth movements might remain constant if our gender roles were reversed, the meanings and perhaps expression of our body language, conversation, and entire relationship would not. As such, our experiences, intersections, and relational narratives can bridge into theoretical discussions of care.

Bridge Two: Spanning Feminist Care Research and Disability Perspectives

The second bridge encourages feminist care scholars to account for disability critiques of care, and disability scholars to consider feminist perspectives. This requires defining care as a tension between competing understandings and includes the critical definitions of care suggested by disability perspectives. This bridge does not aim to include only points of "common ground" (Kröger 2009) and shared "passionate commitments" (Watson et al. 2004, 341) but also (seemingly) irreconcilable insights.

In a scattered, riveting plenary speech, with a rhetorical style that openly reveals the writing process, Margaret Price (2011, 17) explores the idea of practising alliance, as opposed to being an ally. This includes "reflecting upon mistakes – sitting with them – listening to them – [which] is painful," but avoiding wallowing in the privilege of guilt. It is not easy or comfortable to reflect on the oppressive histories and potentials of care, but it is a necessary component to how nondisabled feminist care researchers can practice alliance with disability communities. Creating accessible versions of care is a difficult two-way process in which care researchers seek to engage with disability critiques rather than dismiss them as misguided, and disability scholars equally resist the tendency to condemn feminist care research and theory as "conceptually contaminated" (Kröger 2009, 399).

Killian insists on a relaxed, easygoing approach towards his attendants, reluctant to classify me (or even his paid attendant at the sports tournament) as merely a paid employee. The legacies of institutionalization and the gendered nature of the work are never far removed from Killian; according to him, he aims to take the "institutionalized" approach out of his daily life. The potential for abuse is near the surface, likely contributing to why the most intimate interactions are also the most awkward, as well as to Killian's tendency to hire by personal referral. In addition, Killian often expresses discomfort about asking for assistance, especially unpaid assistance, claiming he does not want to "put people out." This seemingly insignificant yet common reaction is discouraged by Independent Living perspectives that justifiably demand personal support as a right. But at present, most attendant arrangements do not provide all the support a person may require to participate in the diverse activities of life, leaving large gaps that must be filled by relying on unpaid family and friends. As feminist care research shows us, the systemic presumption that informal care will fill in the gaps in public services is typically shorthand for reliance on women, without ensuring that the necessary time, space, and other supports are in place to do this work. Killian's discomfort and reluctance to ask for informal support acknowledge another oppressive side of care, where women and sometimes paid attendants are taken advantage of; required to work in unstable working conditions with few protections and benefits; and at times, though never in our particular example, abused by recipients of care. In this example, we need elements of both disability rejections of care and feminist analysis of care work in order to understand our dynamic.

Bridge Three: Across Divisions within Disability Studies and Communities

The third bridge explores the tensions among disability studies and communities around care in order to move beyond accessibility as a "solution," to create more truly inclusive forms of care. North American society gives primacy to the value of independence (Fineman 2004); it is enshrined in many social policies, legal mechanisms, and even philosophical understandings of personhood (Kittay 2002). The Independent Living movement revises common definitions of independence but still maintains it as an important, if not paramount, social value. In some ways, Independent Living obscures the "inevitable dependencies" of life (Kittay 1999), though it does not eliminate these dependencies as thoroughly as critics of Independent Living imply. In any case, Independent Living includes an emphasis on autonomous decision making, which can be exclusionary towards people who need assistance to make decisions or who do not use verbal communication. Further, there is a well-documented tension between people with physical disabilities and their organizations and people with intellectual impairments, their allies, and organizations (Ryan and Runswick-Cole 2008; Hillyer 1993). Often this tension manifests as a distrust of able-bodied parent advocates and disregard of people with intellectual disabilities. This "hierarchy of impairments," as Deal (2003) terms it, reflects the paradox of valuing self-determination while being physically dependent on the support of an attendant.

At this point, it is useful to incorporate feminist disability theorists' call for ambivalence (Clare 1999; Wendell 1996). Care is full of tension and conflicting messages; as such, it is necessary to approach some of these dilemmas with ambivalence in order to move beyond prevailing political positions and assumptions. Ambivalence provides breathing room by allowing some of the seemingly irresolvable debates to simply remain irresolvable. Ambivalence highlights that no theory is complete – there will always be omissions, oversights, and exceptions in theoretical frameworks. People with disabilities should not be barred from experiences of self-determination, independence, and autonomy; at the same time, independence is not the sole indicator of personhood and success to which some people have access and others do not. Certain feminist care scholars and theorists negotiate this tension via the concept of relational autonomy (Clement 1996). That is, even powerful societal figures who seemingly embody independence and freedom must rely on care and service work to maintain the guise of ultimate autonomy.

The concepts of dependence, autonomy, and interdependence whirl around Killian's and my interactions. We refuse to categorize our relationship as either informal or formal, independent or dependent. The frien-tendant is only sometimes paid, is always a friend, and sometimes does not perform any physical support work at all, and we maintain that the self-manager should be generally in charge of his or her support. Unlike many other care workers, I am not economically dependent on Killian or on a government-funded home care program for my subsistence. But the state and the economy depend on the interactions among Killian, his other attendants, and me to sustain a hidden and increasingly precarious work economy (Vosko 2000) and to enable him to participate in the more visible workforce. In some ways, Killian is also physically dependent on his attendants, and he is left to negotiate his attendant relationships without regular interference or guidance. Our relationship is two-way, and this interdependency is not merely an idiosyncratic trait of our specific relationship. Based on past experiences as an attendant in other contexts,

I also cannot deny that the rhythm of our relationship, including the emphasis on in/ter/dependence, would have a distinctly different tone if Killian had an intellectual disability, particularly if he communicated in nonverbal ways. This does not mean, however, that such an imagined person should be excluded from Independent Living arrangements, as they currently are in certain programs (including the program in this study). Rather, this calls for a more ambivalent positioning on independence to make room for those who cannot attain even revised forms of it.

Bridge Four: From the Local to the Transnational
Creating accessible forms of care extends beyond accounting for people with intellectual disabilities and challenges us to think about how our formulations of care account for transnational links. Independent Living, core disability studies scholarship, and foundational feminist care research largely overlook people with disabilities and support providers in, or who originate from, the Global South (Meekosha 2011). Disability scholarship is only recently beginning to consider movements in the Global South and disability issues from transnational perspectives (e.g., Soldatic 2013; Arenas Conejo 2011; Grech 2011; Erevelles 2011, 2006; Ghai 2002). Robert McRuer (2006, 199 and 204), for example, argues that disability studies are haunted by the "specters of globalization" and must "develop new vocabularies" for discussing varied global bodies. Some of these global bodies are the transnational subjects who travel from the Global South to receive, or more commonly deliver, attendant services in the Global North; significantly, research on Independent Living approaches to attendant services are conspicuously silent on this topic.

According to Robinson (2006), a feminist *political* ethics of care recognizes care as a crucial aspect of healthy and prosperous societies, and frames care as both a private matter and a public concern, in some ways similar to how feminist disability theorists position "disability" (see also Sevenhuijsen 1998; Tronto 1993). For example, Fiona Williams's account (2001) of the political ethics of care identifies varied contemporary forms of care and reveals a complex definition of what counts as care. Williams successfully incorporates disability perspectives, refusing to dismiss them as inconsequential, and Williams's works serves as an example of how the second bridge between care scholars and disability perspectives can operate. The transnationalizing trend Williams (2001, 470) identifies and takes up in her subsequent work (e.g., Williams 2011) is the connection this final bridge seeks to make, as it is essential to consider "geopolitical inequalities between states affecting individuals in gendered and racialized ways" within attendant services. Care is indeed transnational, as indicated by the global migration of care workers (Hondagneu-Sotelo 2007; Zimmerman, Litt, and Bose 2006; Parreñas 2001) and policy frameworks (Ungerson and Yeandle 2007). At present, Independent Living does not provide an adequate framework for analyzing or even documenting this link, making the final bridge more urgent.

The proposal of the feminist political ethics of care is particularly intriguing if it is maintained that care is best understood as an unstable, multifaceted tension between competing meanings. Transforming care into a civic value thus does not mean pulling universal charitable and medical definitions to the centre of social and political conversations, but rather pulling an unstable complexity to the crux of these discussions and perhaps indirectly changing the meanings of civic values. Instead of an abstract sense of justice or an emotional sense of "caring about," social policies can be built on care as an unstable, contradictory category, and can promote a critical reflection on the oppressive legacies and potentials of care.

Disability scholars and activists position personal support as a right. As Krogh (2004, 139) puts it, "Home support [is] a necessary service that mediates citizenship," though arguably this is only a potentiality and not a guarantee of personal assistance. However, these demands are convoluted in a transnational framework. With a variety of examples, Charlton (1998) demonstrates that some of the common tools of disability organizing, such as critiques of charity, are less effective when making more basic demands for services in countries restrained by globally induced debt. Indeed, thinking about the Global South reveals the implicit privilege in our conversations about the language and logistics of attendant services.

How can Killian and I travel across this bridge to the transnational? This bridge requires some difficult stretching, particularly because disability perspectives often focus on the local and experiential. Transnational feminists remind us that such a focus in the Global North can mask our contributions to global inequalities (Erevelles 2011, 2006; Meekosha 2011). To reveal the ways in which our mundane negotiations are connected to these inequalities, it is important to return to the shared social locations identified when speaking about our intersectional experiences. It is not accidental that Killian and I occupy relatively similar shared social locations. Direct-funding models of support, such as the one Killian uses, do not have straightforward protections against employment discrimination, and users express a desire to hire people they can relate to, which often manifests in hiring those with similar cultural backgrounds. Meanwhile, migrant workers increasingly travel across borders and, for one reason or another, end up providing care work. Under direct funding, personal support jobs, which were previously more accessible to immigrant and racialized women, become the purview of postsecondary students. The existence of what Hochschild (2000) terms the "global care chain" dramatically changes how we interpret identities, economies, and the global impacts of directly-funded responses to personal support. These are early insights from a limited viewpoint, and the fourth bridge requires further work, remaining an important area for future exploration.

Closing Thoughts

The bridges built by accessible care do not resolve, or aim to resolve, the contradictions posed by contemporary forms of care that are well documented in academic circles. With these competing trends in mind, it is essential to have a layered definition of care that includes the notion that care can be a form of oppression as well as a critical approach to accessibility that moves beyond "solutions."

Accessible care provides tools for using this unruly definition of care and better equips us for complex discussions of attendant services in particular, and of other care topics in general. No single perspective has all the answers on care in theory or in practice, as I hope the example of Killian and me shows. Our example represents the first bridge, that is, using personal experiences to explore the theoretical. The bridges built by accessible care clear the way to travel back and forth between differing perspectives without having to reject one perspective entirely. This ability helps us work through issues within disability studies, since, without concepts from feminist care theorists such as Kittay (2002) and Clement (1996), it is very difficult to speak about people with intellectual disabilities. Yet, as the fourth bridge reveals, there are risks to focusing too narrowly on the local, as it disguises the ways in which those of us located in the Global North contribute to transnational systems of inequality (Mohanty 2003). Accessible care, and the bridges it builds, offers an important contribution that allows disability and feminist scholars to move beyond both adversarial debate and a focus on common ground to explore attendant services, and other care arrangements and issues, with a multifaceted approach situated in the realities of contemporary globalized socioeconomic systems.

I do not, and will never, provide "care for" Killian. Out of respect for his agency and the contributions of Independent Living, and in light of the history of institutionalization and the ongoing potential for institutionalized approaches to disability, I support or assist him (or whatever term is suggested by disability communities). Ironically, Killian cares about me and his more formal attendants by being aware of "asking too much" and by developing highly responsive relationships with us. Yet, our relationship cannot be interpreted as a simple warm-hearted narrative: there are global implications to enacting a highly individualized, downshifted form of service delivery in a period of accelerated neoliberalism and austerity. We must find ways to acknowledge those whom our relationship displaces, the global bodies who haunt our privileged relationship, and the people with intellectual disabilities who are not eligible for this form of attendant services, in order to demonstrate that accessible practices and conceptualizations of care are indeed (tenuously) possible.

2

Research, Care, and Embracing the Possibilities of Failure

Academic research can be interpreted as a form of care, including all the tensions and complications that concept invokes. Research, like care, can involve conflicting and evolving emotional elements as researchers express passion about, commitment to, and concern for the topics we study. Qualitative research can also involve ambiguous and blurred relationships between researchers and participants, much like the relationships forged between people with disabilities and their attendants. Researchers may adopt a radical social justice framework and approach research as a method of activism, though the broad foundation of social research is a more benevolent aim to illuminate social concerns. Researchers may be implicitly motivated by notions of help, social change, and improvement, similar to what motivates many who choose to enter into caring or helping professions (Christensen 2010; Cushing and Lewis 2002). Like care, the "helping imperative" that undergirds career and personal decisions to engage in research is neither benign nor isolated from ongoing legacies of institutionalization, colonization, and other systems of inequality (Heron 2007). These legacies manifest directly in power-laden interactions between researchers and participants who may occupy divergent social identities, as well as when considering the broader context of the research industry.

Many of the tensions of care, and research, are irresolvable. Researchers, like other care and medical professionals, often occupy positions of power in relation to the participants, although this dynamic is becoming more complex in the neoliberal university. Informed by neoliberal ideologies, the contemporary university in North America includes growing administrative structures and enrolment in graduate programs as well as decreases in tenured faculty positions and high proportions of precariously employed fellows, research associates, and especially contract instructors. This context creates new pressures for emerging researchers to produce results at rates of (or surpassing) tenured faculty in order to "stand out" on the job market. Such precarious researchers now have a substantial, perhaps even dominating, presence in the world at large and collect data amid widely unchallenged societal presumptions about privilege, wealth, and job security that are simply no longer accurate.

Undoubtedly higher education is evolving, but individual research interactions do still include the potential for harm and often a presumed professional status. As Chapman (2012) argues, professional status morally exalts those with formalized credentials, and such exaltation is tethered to the devaluation of marginalized people. The structural injustices of our social and political contexts simultaneously require marginalized people to locate and interact with professionals in order to access programs and services that can be necessary for survival (Kelly and Chapman 2015). This legacy resonates within research dynamics, where nondisabled researchers have been accused of contributing to a "disability industry" that encompasses industrial design, professional services, and social programming geared towards addressing disability in some regard (DePoy and Gilson 2004). In a research context, academics can mobilize "disability" to apply for grants, publish papers, teach courses, and pursue various other professional gains and arguably do so at an accelerated frequency because of the renewed pressures on performance metrics and the highly competitive job market; these activities then form the foundation of a prolific career that does not require accountability to people with disabilities or communities. Erevelles (2014, n.p.) comments on this tension: "It is [community activist] work that has taught me to think with disabilities and it would be remiss of me to not acknowledge the generosity of their labor that is sometimes appropriated by credentialed academics with little acknowledgement or recognition of the conditions within which this knowledge was produced." The reality of life for disabled activists, and for disabled people more generally, may not always be reflected in disability research. Individual researchers may elect to practice reflexivity or attempt to work with and gain credibility from disability communities, but such activities are not necessary to succeed professionally in the neoliberal academy.

The relative power and prestige resulting from participating in the academy and presenting oneself to the world as a researcher does not go unnoticed from those outside the system. Many potential research participants refuse to participate if they are suspicious of the researcher's ability to create a legitimate representation or if they disagree with the framework of the proposed study. Alternatively, some research participants are motivated to draw on the (presumed) social capital the researcher has, implicitly or explicitly granting authority to the researcher to use their narratives in productive and potentially transformative ways that will improve their lives, or the lives of others. Undoubtedly, the researcher-researched relationship presents a complex, power-laden dynamic that must be approached with openness and caution. This chapter enters at this point, in order to explore the research process as a critical form of care that requires vigilance to avoid potential abuse. The research process, however, will always include failures. Seeing failure as possibility will help recognize the systemic structures of dominance that research industry and individual researchers operate within.

This chapter explores tensions of research in an attempt to practice feminist reflexivity and to demonstrate the complexities of care. The methods and specificities of this project are examples in a larger conversation about research dynamics, structural inequalities, and the role of emotion in work. While recounting the stages of research, I include moments of impasse, difficult questions, and hesitations. As the exploration of these moments show, qualitative research is presented as messy, irregular, and rife with dilemmas. Further, these dilemmas are not isolated incidents of discomfort but can be situated within a broader context of an academic research industry that has its own histories (and ongoing practices) of oppression, hierarchy, and contributions to social inequalities.

Autoethnography

The first bridge of accessible care argues that care is a visceral, relational, and experiential practice that demands lived reflection to make sense of theoretical questions. Autoethnography is a method where "the researcher uses personal lived experiences as the primary source of ethnographic data" (Buch and Staller 2007, 189). In this study, my experiences were treated as one source of supplementary data. Autoethnography reflects the values of feminist standpoint epistemology, where situated and partial knowledges, typically from marginalized perspectives, offer a more accurate and, some argue, objective view of the world (Collins 2009; Haraway 1988). Autoethnography is also an avenue for self-reflexivity and gestures towards the techniques of influential scholars and allied scholars in disability studies. I do not identify as disabled and largely do not occupy a "voice from the margins," as promoted in feminist standpoint epistemology. Yet, it remains important to locate myself within the research to help reveal the limitations, potentials, and mechanisms of the research industry.

My impetus for researching disability and attendant services stems from personal reflection on former employment as an attendant in differing settings, observing friends who employ attendants, and prior research on models of support provision. Like many care workers, I came to attendant work as a young person naively motivated by a desire to help, or perhaps with what disabled activists would term a "caring" orientation. Such motivations, particularly those that remain in the realm of benign, apolitical community service, are strongly encouraged among Canadian youth, to the extent that the Ontario Ministry of Education requires high school students to complete forty hours of volunteer work in order to graduate. This becomes complicated, as Kennelly (2011, 2) aptly observes, when individual motivation transforms from notions of "good citizen" towards social justice and confrontational activism, where youth are "vilified as irrational, violent, and out-of-control."

My approach to disability was transformed from one that was charitable and caring to one rooted in social justice through my experiences of living in a L'Arche community. L'Arche is a global network of intentional communities for people with intellectual disabilities that grew out of deinstitutionalization. The communities have a spiritual and at times religious orientation, which attendants and community members do not have to participate in (Kelly 2010). At L'Arche, I lived and worked with people who did not speak, move, or eat in conventional ways. L'Arche claims to be apolitical in terms of advocacy directed at the government. With a wider understanding of politics (Angrosino 2003), L'Arche is a unique response to disability that is not medical or institutionalized, and values people with varied capabilities as contributing members in a diverse community. I slowly reconfigured my own understandings of disability through relationships, physically assisting people with their daily needs, maintaining our shared household, and the difficult process of confronting my assumptions. The first days were spent observing and learning, as L'Arche makes space for those who need assistance to become comfortable with new attendants before they are offered hands-on assistance. I felt awkward and uncomfortable as I stared at both the attendants and the individuals with profound physical and intellectual disabilities. On my first day, I was particularly uneasy about one young woman who was eating lunch through a tube that ran directly into her stomach. I sat still during lunch, unsure of where to look or what to think. Over a very short period, this mode of eating transformed to something normal and everyday, and it was a task I comfortably assisted with. I look back at my ignorant and perhaps dehumanizing approach to the people I met, an approach that transitioned into meaningful, complicated relationships and a desire to challenge misguided worldviews. I arrived at L'Arche motivated by what Heron (2007) terms the "helping imperative," striving towards Kennelly's notion of good citizen (2011), but I left engaged and with concrete evidence that a different response to disability is possible.

After L'Arche, I had other experiences as an attendant and came to the broader world of disability by completing graduate work in disability studies and forging relationships with people with varied disabilities, including my partner. For my master's research I studied L'Arche and Independent Living, as models demonstrating different approaches to disability. The research questions for this project, however, crystallized after thinking about Killian, a close friend who uses the Direct Funding Program. I had assisted him before and observed his interactions with attendants prior to starting this study. Killian knows he is often my reference point when I work through complex ideas, and he figures in other parts of this book.

Although adding to a rich and transparent description of research, auto-ethnography carries a unique set of challenges. Before the research began, I was confronted with my first ethical dilemma: Were my observations and inter-actions with Killian mine? His? Ours? I asked permission from Killian to write about him but continue to struggle with how to represent him fairly. He deeply informs this work, and it would be unfair to leave him out; yet, it is unfair to include him when it is my voice and not his that narrates. Ellis (2007, 16–17) grapples with the many ethical dilemmas of research that arise outside "pro-cedural ethics"; she argues, "To write an effective autoethnography demands showing perceived warts and bruises as well as the accolades and successes." But such an approach violates the basic agreements of friendships when auto-ethnographic accounts include interactions with other people. As the feminist ethics of care shows us, we live relationally and interdependently (Clement 1996; Gilligan 1982). An autoethnographic account does not represent a disconnected voice that navigates and responds to the world independently, but will encompass relationships and interactions with a range of others. The challenge lies in handling this dynamic without replicating the history of a disembodied and location-less researcher speaking for others, especially if the researcher occupies a place of privilege in relation to those in the accounts.

In our conversations, Killian and I joke about our ethically questionable relationship. He seems at ease, trusting, and light in these conversations, but under the laughter I am tense about violating an imaginary set of research rules. I was reluctant and nervous to show him my writing at first, despite his ongoing interest in the project. What would he think? Was I slipping into what Haraway (1988) terms the "godtrick," or a complex, subtle form of ventriloquism as Michelle Fine (1992) describes? I continually fret over these ethical, relational, and representational conundrums, tentatively making decisions and waiting for the inevitable slips I will make. No formula exists for approaching these situations. Approaching these situations through autoethnography and treating research dilemmas as pertinent and valuable data will not always succeed in addressing the complex challenges inherent in qualitative research. At times, however, this approach may challenge and transform the experience of research for both participants and researchers. If such experiences are replicated, encouraged, and multiplied, perhaps we can tentatively head towards an "opening" of the parameters of research without, as Shotwell (2012) warns in the context of social change, abandoning the need to maintain normativities and standards in our work.

What is it about Killian that informs this study in such a foundational way? He appears to live an independent life, supported by a vibrant network of attendants who he has carefully cultivated over a decade. While using and thoroughly endorsing an Independent Living model of attendant services, he and his network of attendants simultaneously reflect feminist writing about interdependency (e.g., Arneil 2009; Fine and Glendinning 2005; Clement 1996; Gilligan 1982). Further, my own experiences living and then researching L'Arche reveals that these communities *require* meaningful relationships to operate (Kelly 2010; Cushing and Lewis 2002). But these observations do not signify a failure or inadequacy of Independent Living. Rather, Killian, his attendants, and L'Arche reveal an important fissure in the documented debates among disability and feminist scholars on the understanding of care. Like Clement (1996, 24) describes, these examples demonstrate that "relationships, and specifically caring relationships, are a necessary precondition for autonomy."

Autoethnography recounts a world of people, openly revealing the effect of the researcher on the results and how relationships undergird and sustain a seemingly autonomous worldview. This research process reflects the ways in which relationships with, and assistance from, an attendant can enable a person with a disability to participate more freely in the world, both autonomously and with others. Through and beyond the autoethnographic reflections, it is clear that the notions of interdependence and independence are not mutually exclusive or in competition, but rather are in conversation.

On Finding Each Other and Forging Relationships

Yoshida et al.'s account (2000) of the history of Ontario's Direct Funding Program document the different political figures, nonprofit groups, and individuals involved in the formation and ongoing administration of the program. As such, beyond autoethnography, for this study I interviewed key informants who represent these sectors: public servants, politicians, community advocates, and people working in the daily administration of the program at Independent Living centres. I also analyzed written material from government and community sources in order to document the public, formal narratives on the Direct Funding Program and individualized funding more broadly.

Recruiting the key informants went fairly smoothly. I contacted the Centre for Independent Living in Toronto for recommendations and used a snowball recruitment technique, which resulted in nineteen key informants. I initially told them that they would not be anonymous, in order to encourage them to speak from their official roles. As the research progressed, I elected to mask the identities of these key informants in academic publications because the categories for recruitment often overlapped. Certain key informants were also self-managers and would talk about their own experiences with Direct Funding, which complicated their perspectives as public figures and challenged the university ethics category of vulnerable populations. Early on in the interview process, the topic of individualized funding – a separate advocacy movement led by people with intellectual disabilities and their allies – arose and I began asking for materials and referrals to people working in this area. It was necessary to explore how the push for individualized funding evolved (and remains) distinct from efforts surrounding the Direct Funding Program, despite obvious similarities. I conducted the majority of the forty-five- to ninety-minute interviews in person, making several trips to Toronto and other parts of Ontario.

One particular telephone conversation while recruiting key informants stands out as a pivotal point in the research. One community advocate and past program administrator was difficult to contact. I left many messages by phone and email, and we finally connected over the phone. The potential participant was very upset, yelling angrily at me. He admonished me for exploring care and even advocacy in my research materials. "We don't need care!" and "We [Independent Living] are not allowed to do advocacy!" he proclaimed. The tension gradually dissipated as I outlined my history of involvement with disability organizations and issues, a practice required to varying degrees in my interactions with disability advocates. I convinced him that I was interested in whether "care" was still as controversial as it once was, and that I was fully aware of the disability critiques of this concept. The conversation ended amicably, and he agreed to be interviewed for the study.

This conversation had a few lasting effects on the research. First and foremost, I downplayed the term "care" in the research materials, mentioning it only once in the letter of information so as not to offend potential participants before even starting. When meeting with the participants, I asked directly about care – but only much later in the interview and framed as a matter of semantics. Second, this conversation encouraged me to use my own experiences to increase the level of trust, though I continue to feel uneasy about references to my partner's identity as a disabled person and my volunteer involvements. Most substantially, however, this conversation cast doubt on academic literature claiming that the tensions between disability and feminist perspectives on care are lessening or heading towards resolution. Rather, the incident with this participant is evidence that care remains a highly provocative concept within the Direct Funding Program. The critiques of care brought forth by disability perspectives in and out of the academy cannot be theorized out of existence, dismissed as unimportant, or erased by grouping attendant services with other forms of home care. This pivotal confrontation demonstrated how important it is to take the disability critiques of care seriously, a premise that undergirds the theoretical concept of accessible care and the overall approach of this book. Research must be approached as a form of care, including all the tensions that "care" evokes, and this encounter reveals the types of presumptions a researcher can replicate, sustaining knowledge and truths in theoretical and academic spheres that do not reflect the experiences of those using, working, and designing the programs. Further, such knowledge can promulgate without question, gaining authority and propelling research careers. In light of this particular conversation, it became necessary to reconsider the study's approach as a mechanism to reveal the critical tensions of care and research.

With a new approach in hand, I proceeded to organize a second set of interviews with fourteen self-managers (plus six key informants who were also self-managers), fifteen attendants, and six informal supports. Feminist ethics of care are grounded in daily experiences of giving and receiving support, whereas feminist disability scholars value personal narratives, making these interviews an integral reflection of the theoretical framework of this study. I started the interviews with Killian, who was proactive and eager, and the formal research was completed quickly. Even though I was fumbling and somewhat rigid with my questions during our first interview, Killian's responses were eloquent, and I knew our previously established rapport contributed to the interview's success. I learned to be less "professional" during these interviews, which often took place in the homes of the participants or coffee shops and took between sixty and ninety minutes. I conducted thirty- to forty-minute follow-up interviews with a few attendants, and with almost all the self-managers. Outside our interview, Killian quickly passed on contact information for his attendants and informal supports, and spoke to them directly to encourage participation. We frequently joked about the difficulty in maintaining confidentiality, as he was curious to know what his attendants and informal supports were saying to me and how the research was going. Killian and I are still friends, and he continued to inquire about the research long after the data collection was completed. I cannot overemphasize the support and encouragement he provided throughout the entire process.

Although the importance of developing rapport and forming a variety of relationships in an ethnographic field is well documented and discussed in most introductory methods textbooks, there is little methodological literature on including previously established friends as participants, with notable exceptions (Taylor 2011; Tillmann-Healy 2003). Taylor (2011, 11) discusses the benefits of already established rapport, commenting that "formal interviews are augmented by ongoing opportunities to talk with and observe [intimate informants] in moments that are significant yet often random and unexpected – moments that one is only privy to as a result of intimate contact." As with all relationships, research participants are often more willing to share their insights and recount highly personal experiences when there is an established fondness towards the researcher that extends beyond professional rapport. Further, including friends as research participants allows for a complex form of reciprocity developed over an extended period in variable ways, rather than by directly providing honorariums or other arrangements. But Taylor (2011, 15) also recommends a "mix of intimately familiar and unfamiliar informants" in order to avoid the pitfalls of an insular study. In this particular study, including intimate informants in some ways replicates the ambiguous relationships that form between attendants and people with disabilities, relationships that tread across formal/informal, professional/friend boundaries. In direct-funding arrangements, people with disabilities often hire friends to work as attendants or become friends with their attendants in an attempt to reduce risk and maintain a sense of home by building on or establishing a relationship (Kietzman, Benjamin, and Matthias 2008; Matthias and Benjamin 2008; Whitlach and Feinberg 2006). This approach to attendants can create awkwardness and ambiguity regarding working conditions, expected norms of interaction, and perhaps even romantic tensions intertwined with physical and financial consequences. Including friend-participants provides access to the ethical dilemmas attendants and self-managers may face by requiring the researcher to engage in somewhat similar relational ambiguities.

After Killian, I had difficulties with recruitment for this phase. I presumed more self-managers would know each other, but I found that the participants in this study were busy and somewhat disconnected from one another. After finding only two participants using the snowball technique, I opened the study to anyone in Ontario. I also included three other friends as participants. Because of privacy concerns, the Centre for Independent Living in Toronto was not able to send out an email on my behalf, which was understandable in light of the history of outsider research on people with disabilities. I ended up contacting people through other disability organizations, though I had little response from mass emails. I also contacted the local Independent Living Centres in Ottawa and Kingston and thereby found two participants. My spouse comes across people with disabilities through his work and participation in adaptive sport and referred two participants to the study. Eventually, Killian sent out personalized emails to people on a private contact list from the Centre for Independent Living in Toronto. This was Killian's idea, and it rounded up three more participants.

In short, recruitment was slow and difficult, and much more complex than I had initially anticipated. On four occasions, I conducted an interview with a self-manager, but either he or she would not pass on attendant contact information or the attendant was unwilling to participate. On three occasions, attendants did not want to participate because of language concerns (i.e., English was not their first language), revealing a substantial limitation of this study. The attendants are an elusive group of people, unaffiliated with each other or formal organizations and most often working for only one self-manager. As for the informal supports, although the number of participants is low, many self-managers insisted they were not reliant on informal supports at this point in their lives. There was some tension around this insistence, as participants also reported not having enough hours and detailed strategies for finding extra help. All the participants are given pseudonyms, and Killian has two so that he does not stand out in later chapters.

I was the most confident and the process was the quickest with participants with whom I had an established relationship, perhaps reflecting the natural rhythm Tillmann-Healy (2003) suggests in her "friendship as method" approach. Yet, our interactions were not completely natural. A formality was signified by the use of a digital recorder, scripted questions for the first few participants (until I felt confident to interview without the guide), and my taking notes. Regardless of prior relationships, many participants seemed to prefer a formal interview, where I asked a question and the participant responded directly, as opposed to a more conversational interview. This was surprising in light of the focus in feminist research approaches on levelling power imbalances. Michelle Fine and colleagues (2000, 115) offer a possible explanation:

Many of the women and men we interviewed both recognized and delight-
fully exploited the power inequalities in the interview process. They recognized that we could take their stories, their concerns, and their worries to
audiences, policy makers, and the public in ways that they themselves could
not, because they would not be listened to.

Many, and perhaps most, of the participants in this phase of the research saw
the interview as an opportunity to voice concerns and potentially improve the
Direct Funding Program and thereby improve the lives of both the self-managers
and attendants. The participants were aware that research is an industry that
includes access to power and were invested in maintaining the authority implied
by this industry.

I was not friends with the majority of participants, and still would not categorize our relationships in these terms. It is important to respect and engage
deeply with people who participate in research projects, and the points of established friendship proved particularly fruitful, but I am not convinced that
progressive research should demand forming close relationships with all participants. This sometimes seems like the logical extension of discussions about
the importance of rapport within anti-oppressive research.

One complication with friendship in the research process is the tension
between "trustworthiness and reciprocity" (Harrison, MacGibbon, and Morton
2001) – that is, meeting standards of credibility in the research community
while maintaining relationships and honouring the words of the participants.
These aims are not always mutually exclusive, though there are moments that
require discretion and ethical consideration. It is difficult to deal with contradictions and negative statements from friend-participants when the natural
inclination is to protect the relationship by focusing on unproblematic elements.
Further, there is the issue of never-ending consent, which I experienced with
Killian, as his trust in me is so great that he never declines if I ask to include
something in the research (see also Bhattacharya 2007).

Garton and Copland (2010) suggest that prior relationships require a complex negotiation of roles in an interview setting, and that this process poses
more difficulties for the interviewer than for the participant. Yet, in the study,
this process provided an opportunity for some participants to take central roles
and for others to be less involved. Reflecting on my data-collection experience,
I realize that the conventional definition of "key informant" is not accurate. In
this project, instead of being official public figures with authoritative viewpoints,
key informants are central participants who are deeply involved in the entire
research process, echoing a participatory action approach (Dick 2009; Herr and

Anderson 2005). It is essential for these people to directly or indirectly indicate a high level of interest and availability in order to avoid unnecessary burden on them and to ensure participation of other people who may not want such a level of involvement. An opportunity can be presented to these self-identified participants to become more involved, but such involvement is not mandatory for the project to proceed. Making space for this new type of key informant is one method of acknowledging research as a form of care with tensions and unequal allocations of authority. Such an approach requires the researcher to reconsider his or her worldview, role, and need to control the outcomes, and hinges on the key informant outlining the aspects he or she would like to contribute to. This flexible approach allows for friendships to (sometimes) develop or be drawn on, degrees of participation, and a reciprocal accountability that is not overly taxing on participants.

Role of the Researcher: Where "In" Ends and "Out" Begins

My partner, as I've mentioned, has a physical disability, and recently we started using minimal semi-private attendant services for assistance around the house. The service we use sent four different attendants over four weeks. I understand care as a relationship, albeit a tense one, but in reality, up until this point there has not been an opportunity to cultivate relationships with the attendants. Further, one of these attendants actively resisted interacting with us by talking on her phone the entire time she was at our house. Undoubtedly, the structure of service delivery greatly affects the potential for relationships, the working conditions for attendants, and the quality of the services delivered. The model we use does not include the option to hire or choose which attendants come to assist us. On a personal level, I grappled with my expectations of privacy and with the question of whether we deserved help – and these attendants were not even assisting me or my husband with personal care needs. This is a new experience for us, one we are still navigating, and it is starkly different from my previous work experience as an attendant in various settings.

My academic work leads me to read, write, and teach about disability, gender, and care based on past employment and research, family members with disability, and ongoing involvement as a volunteer in disability-related organizations. So am I in or am I out? An eloquent, in-depth film review boils down to "worth seeing or not worth seeing" and, similarly, although academics write about degrees of insider/outsider status (Hesse-Biber 2007), everyday experiences of research presents a simple yes or no question. I was regarded with ambivalence and even hostility by some research participants, even when I was open about my position in the world. As mentioned, at one frustrating point, Killian used his insider status to canvass on my behalf and recruit participants. Throughout the research process, I have been acutely aware of my outsider label. I can claim to live with disability, but I am not disabled. I am not trying to avoid a stigmatized label or imply that disability is something different from me, but I do want to avoid co-opting a marginalized identity to which I do not feel entitled. Claiming a disabled identity (assuming such a claim would be accepted) would not challenge the notions of insider/outsider. Alternatively, McRuer (2006, 34) dismantles the binary categories of disabled and nondisabled in order to explore "what it might mean to come out crip" (see also Schalk 2013). This coming out is not reserved for bodies traditionally categorized as disabled but is open to bodies and cultural applications that disrupt and interrogate the status quo – for example, disabled and queer bodies. As such, McRuer, like other queer theorists, attempts to move beyond the limits of identity politics. This radical perspective has yet to infiltrate many social justice groups and individual political positioning. Further, the foundations of crip theory and other post-identity theories may not be able to immediately and effectively ameliorate the many material disadvantages experienced by marginalized people. Although the radical potential of coming out crip is intriguing, I remain uncomfortable with claiming such a perspective in public and community forums where it may not be understood. I relate to Erevelles's assertion (2014, n.p.): "My complicated status as outsider/outsider-within makes me thoughtfully cautious of any attempts to make definite sense of these borderlands."

I am openly "out" about my varied roles and clearly "in" this book. I engage with autoethnography to reflect my blurred position between in and out, and the potentials and limits of identifying as an ally. In feminist disability studies, there is a preference towards writing from personal experiences of disability, or what Garland-Thomson (2002) terms "sitpoint epistemology" (see also Kimpson 2005; Lindgren 2004; Titchkosky 2003; Linton 1998; Mairs 1996). This draws on the tradition of feminist standpoint epistemology (Collins 2009; Naples 2003a) or "situated knowledge" that presumes "only partial perspective promises objective vision" (Haraway 1988, 583). This is distinctly different from writing from the role of an ally. In disability studies, it is less common to endorse allied positions in research and theorizing, likely because of the tendency to "speak for" disabled people who have been so often spoken for throughout history. Price and Shildrick (2002, 64) comment: "It is as though there is a reluctance [in disability studies] to acknowledge that someone without evident disabilities could have anything useful to say, or at the most her role would be strictly subsidiary." There is a profound "danger of romanticizing and/or appropriating the vision of the less powerful while claiming to see from their positions" (Haraway 1988, 584). Yet, particularly for someone who sits on the precarious edge of insider/outsider and attempts to "practice alliance" (Price 2011), I hope to add something to the conversation.

Some disability scholars who are also parents of people with disabilities present compelling analyses from their positions as allies (Bérubé 2010, 1998; Douglas 2010b; Kittay 2010, 1999; Ryan and Runswick-Cole 2008; Hillyer 1993), and feminist disability studies makes room for ambivalence (Clare 1999; Wendell 1997). It is important to be cautious and sensitive to our essentialist tendencies and weary of "speaking for another," but we cannot shut down the conversation that emerges from the complex engagements with our shifting, conflicting identities and relationships. Lennard Davis (1995, xvii) claims to write partly from "that in-between liminal position I occupied and still occupy" as a child of Deaf parents. As Hillyer (1993, 107) concludes her chapter on mother-blaming, "The politics of disability are incomplete without our hearing also the stories of nondisabled people who nevertheless live with disability." That is to say, allies to people with disabilities, particularly close allies (e.g., family members, life partners, even long-term attendants) also have understandings of disability. These viewpoints are not the same as experiencing and identifying as disabled, but they have the potential to contribute to the conversations. Such an approach must proceed with caution and delicacy, as the pull towards dominating, coercive forms of care and research will perpetually exist.

As feminist ethics of care scholars demonstrate, we are interdependent and live through relationships. In some of the earliest ethics of care scholarship, Gilligan (1982, 29) argues that the women in her studies see "a world comprised of relationships rather than of people standing alone, a world that coheres through human connection rather than through systems of rules," and that this awareness is the basis for an alternative mode of moral decision making that contrasts abstract models of justice. Decisions are made and knowledge is created through and in reference to relationships (see also Lugones and Spelman 1983). Qualitative research as a knowledge-generating enterprise can perhaps be understood, then, in terms of relational standpoints between researchers and participants, rather than in terms of insider/outsider statuses. Knowledge about disability, care, and programs such as Direct Funding is created in the interactions between attendants and self-managers. The challenge is how to capture this space while writing independently, a challenge I do not have a simple solution for.

Analysis and Representation

What happens between qualitative data collection and the final written product is often veiled by what Doucet (2006) terms a "gossamer wall" between researcher and readers. It is difficult to explain qualitative data analysis, since much of it is intuitive and builds on the prior knowledge and insights of the researcher. I attempt to capture the messages about care, and the practical relevance of these messages, through my interpretation of what was created during the interviews and what is conveyed through the documents. In writing, I attempt to explain my thoughts and gesture towards other studies that may confirm or refute these interpretations.

For this project, I began by using NVivo, software designed for qualitative data analysis. These types of programs aid the researcher in breaking down and classifying large amounts of information, almost beyond recognition. When using this program, researchers can overlook the context central to qualitative analysis. The program attempts to quantify the unquantifiable and can easily cause the researcher to miss both passing details and complex examples that do not easily fit into categories. But passing details might not have general significance, and sweeping conclusions are not the point of qualitative research. On the other hand, the software does provide a starting point for the daunting process of sorting through large amounts of information. My analysis also includes handwritten notes and diagrams, related and unrelated journal articles, news stories, and books. Through these varied sources, I began to make connections that often sprung up unexpectedly. For example, the idea for the theoretical framework of accessible care came not only from reading about care for many years but also from reflecting on the phone conversation I had with the participant who was upset with me for using the word "care." That conversation reminded me that, despite recent academic literature suggesting that "the fundamental conceptual antagonism between care research and disability studies seems to have become diluted recently" (Kröger 2009, 406), in Ontario it is still a highly loaded, and even offensive, word for some. I could not just forge ahead with my use of the term but had to change it to make it inclusive, or accessible, for people with disabilities – or else avoid using it all together.

I had (and still have) deep hesitations about using the highly critical tools of academic accountability on (against?) the disability community, Killian, and the other participants. It can be difficult to achieve a balance between these two aims, particularly when less-than-flattering insights emerge. Ellis infamously returned to the fishing communities she had studied for many years through active participant observation to find the participants felt betrayed and offended by her work once it was published. She recounts: "When I returned to Fishneck, my friends there confronted me with the words I had written" (2007, 11). As well as describing the participants, it is necessary to consider how to represent the people whom they represent in their narratives. This dilemma is what Michelle Fine and colleagues (2000) refer to as the "triple representational problem," that is, how to represent ourselves, the participants, and the "others" – people who do not participate but are evoked by the participants, often in hurtful ways. In this study, I could choose to present surface-level but constructive critiques of the Direct Funding Program (Spandler 2004) or choose to engage with some of the more troubling elements, such as the exclusion of people with intellectual disabilities and often-hurtful comments about these people and their allies.

Fine and colleagues (2000, 119–20) urge researchers to "refrain from the naïve belief that these voices should stand on their own or that voices should (or do) survive without theorizing." It is important to include the potentially hurtful elements of analysis but also to pull them away from individuals. This extends to contradictions and errors in information, as it is not the purpose of qualitative interviews to catch participants making mistakes (Portelli 1991). Researchers must also avoid imagining meanings not intended, for example, "repoliticizing perspectives narrated by people who have tried hard to represent themselves as nonpolitical" (Fine et al. 2000, 218). This came into play when I asked participants about their relationship to the Independent Living movement. Quite a few participants saw Direct Funding as just another means to the end of attendant services, albeit a much better means than other options, and claimed to have no opinion on Independent Living as a social movement.

Some scholars suggest the strategy of "respondent validation" or "member checking" at this phase, or earlier phases, to help address issues of representation (Hesse-Biber 2007; Maxwell 2005). I did so in previous research (Kelly 2010) and found that the majority of participants were uninterested in making further contributions of time. It is important to be cognizant and careful when writing and analyzing words that come from another's standpoint, particularly when those words emerge at the urging of and in relationship with the researcher. The participants, however, cannot do this delicate work for the researcher. Nor is the answer to promote "insider" research; a sense of a shared identity may initially open doors, but it is highly fluid and "can change even in the course of a single interview" (Hesse-Biber 2007, 143). Representing other people through academic writing is a calculated gamble and will be refuted and perhaps misrepresentative in certain instances. A researcher's account, whether it is "member checked" or stands alone, offers only a partial viewpoint. Acknowledging the potential for harm is the crux of academic writing, and of seeing research as a form of care.

Closing Thoughts

Qualitative research, like care, can be an all-encompassing process requiring vigilant awareness of power on the part of the researcher and constant reflection on choices and assumptions. In many ways, all research encompasses failure, as projects will never unfold as we originally envision them. There will be unexpected implications for the empirical findings, the communities we claim to represent, and the varied relationships we form with participants. The challenge thus lies in holding and exploring our failures, and it is paramount to acknowledge that care *is also* a form of oppression among other meanings. Patty Douglas (2010b) calls attention to how notions of failure circulate around education, mothering, and disability. The failures of care, like the failures of research, do not signify an ending but represent ongoing possibilities to build relationships, enable flourishing, and create alternative ontologies. The humbling practice of confronting research as failure heads towards renewed academic practices and norms. Such norms are paradoxically disruptive to the standard research protocol, challenging us beyond self-reflection to explore the complex and at times troubling consequences of the research process.

The methodological choices, such as autoethnography, including friends as participants, qualitative analysis, and interviews, do not necessarily apply to other research, even on similar topics. Yet the reflexive *process* that seeks to find, hold, and openly share research failures and successes can begin to address larger questions of social injustice. Whether we openly engage in this process or not, individual research projects are part of a larger research industry, complete with intended and unintended social and individual impacts. Research is a part of the dominant social structures, yet there is potential to frame research as a disruptive intervention and a possible form of resistance.

PART 2

Removing Care

3

"In My Mind That's Not What Care Is"
Care Is Not What Happens Here

Independent Living encompasses a philosophy of disability, complete with specific terminology and an inversion of power dynamics, that is different from medical and social service understandings of disabled people as passive patients or clients. Building on this philosophical commitment, it also encompasses alternative policy mechanisms for long-term care and home care that centre on the person with a disability. Under Independent Living, disabled people direct the actions of the attendants and take control over their interactions, which contrasts the approach of the "care professional," who makes decisions on the behalf of service users. In short, Independent Living is markedly different from other forms of home care; it is so distinct, that it is not care. The messaging is clear in the academic literature and among activist groups, and often in public material from Independent Living centres. This chapter explores to what extent a similar orientation is expressed by the diverse standpoints of the key informants and within the daily interactions between self-managers and attendants in the localized setting of Ontario's Direct Funding Program.

When asked if he sees himself as providing care while working as a Direct Funding attendant, Adam states: "With [the self-manager,] it's more like I'm just helping him out. In my mind that's not what care is. Of course it is, but it's probably my own personal ideas about what that word means." The distancing from care does not seem to be only Adam's personal ideas, as his attitude reflects a rejection of care influenced by Independent Living philosophy and disability studies. These ideas show up in attendant interactions and descriptions of these interactions in the specific contexts of the Direct Funding Program. Several questions arise, however: What makes attendant services different from other forms of care? What definitions of care are operating in the highly localized settings of direct-funding interactions? The attendants and self-managers presumably care about each other in an emotional and relational sense, so what concepts are substituted to describe these components of their daily interactions?

Generally, care is not what happens "here" within the Direct Funding Program or attendant services more broadly, a sentiment encapsulated in Adam's statement. There is also a conflicted and convoluted sense of what care *is*. According to the participants, care has multiple elements, some of which are consistently condemned, while others must happen and may even be appropriate in attendant services. The inclusions of care surrounding the program are explored in the next chapter.

Care encompasses too much and not enough to describe what is happening under Direct Funding. Exploring aspects of the daily interactions between attendants and self-managers creates a reference for "non-care." Garland-Thomson (1997) and other disability theorists demonstrate that disability becomes a reference point for defining "normal" and, similarly, establishing what is "not care" will allude to what remains of it. The rejection of care circulates while it is simultaneously permitted, demonstrating another example of how care can be interpreted as a tension.

Accounts of daily interactions make it clear that attendants play multiple roles. However, two dominant descriptions emerge: attendants as "arms and legs" and attendants as relationship workers. The "arms and legs" role refers to the tangible tasks of attendant work, done under the direction of the self-manager. This direction can veer into the language of automation and creates varied senses of responsibility among the attendants. The relational work between self-managers and attendants remains "not care," in spite of the emotional and interpersonal elements of the descriptions. Relational work is freely spoken about, difficult to describe and negotiate, and mandatory; it also can become inappropriate. The relational work is skilled yet distinct from the sociological concept of emotional labour. One example of a specific technique of this work: the more experienced attendants develop a chameleon personality while self-managers reportedly leave room for attendants to exercise agency, thereby creating relational epistemologies and ontologies between attendants and self-managers. Although in some ways these two dominant descriptions reflect the feminist distinction between caring for and caring about (Grant et al. 2004; Finch and Groves 1983), it is significant that many participants insist this is not care.

Before presenting the activities and descriptions that are "not care," let us return to the first and second bridges of accessible care. The latter is the bridge between feminist perspectives and disability perspectives on care. This bridge compels us to see multiple points of view, and to understand how a person may embody these sometimes conflicting perspectives at any given moment. This bridge is reflected in the scholarly inclusions of feminist and disability literatures and, more tangibly, in the inclusion of recipients, providers, and a few informal supports as participants. Further, there are limited themes exclusive to attendants or self-managers in this study, as the comments can be viewed alongside each other and occasionally against each other. Including varied scholarly and participant voices helps present a fuller picture of Direct Funding. Inclusions of multiple perspectives reflect the disability studies notion that we are all temporarily able-bodied (e.g., L. Davis 2002), and the idea that disability is a pervasive cultural category (Garland-Thomson 2002), implying that anyone can potentially contribute to discussions of disability. Yet, including diverse voices also respects the feminist notion of standpoint epistemologies that suggest that individuals occupy unique social locations with distinct outlooks on the world (e.g., Collins 2009; Naples 2003a, 2003b; or "sitpoint epistemology" as reclaimed by Garland-Thomson 2002). The focus on narratives and interactions stems from the first bridge of accessible care, that is, the use of daily experiences to explore theoretical questions.

Care: A "Bad Four-Letter Word"

For many, "care" remains somewhat of a "bad word, [a] bad four-letter word" as Frank, a self-manager, comments. Some of the self-managers and attendants, and many of the key informants, made clear attempts to distance attendant services from care. The message was strong: forty-two of the fifty-four participants had, with varying degrees of urgency, concerns with the term "care." Numerous participants did not seem to mind the word itself but expressed elements of the Independent Living critiques of care in other parts of the conversation. Of the twelve participants who seemed unaware and unconcerned about the tensions around care, five were informal supports and thus a step away from the Direct Funding Program.

Jennifer, a community advocate and self-manager, describes how she views Independent Living and care as being diametrically opposed and suggests that the concept of care is irredeemable:

> *Jennifer:* I see them as diametrically opposed. So I think that [academic care researchers] don't really understand what Independent Living is all about if they need to bring the term "care" into it.

CK: But some talk about changing the meaning, though; they don't talk about bringing what we think of as care, but sort of reclaiming care is the idea.

Jennifer: Yeah ... no. That doesn't work for me. There's just too much toothpaste out of the tube on that one.

CK: Too much baggage?

Jennifer: Yeah, exactly, too much baggage. Too many associations with the term "care" to be able to redefine it. It's like, "Let's redefine what 'red' means." Everyone knows what red is as a colour. Red is red. But you're not going to say that "red is the new purple." You're going to spend so much time explaining what you mean and don't mean by "care."

Jennifer's position implies that it is easy to define care – red is red, and care is care – and that this is simply not what is happening in Independent Living models of support. The "toothpaste" Jennifer refers to are the multifaceted forms of oppression linked to care. When asked directly, Jennifer says that care is care, and for her that means it is clearly a form of oppression targeting people with disabilities. Care, for Jennifer – and for Adam too, as evidenced by his statement cited earlier – encompasses too much to describe attendant services, which involves help with daily needs and nothing more.

It was easier for interviewees to describe care as happening *somewhere else* than to describe what is actually different about personal assistance. Mathieu, an attendant with many years of experience, describes the other settings he works in:

Mathieu: [outside Direct Funding] I have a, a private client who I take care of. Well I say "take care" because it feels more like I'm doing at-home nursing for him.

CK: It doesn't feel like attendant care, is that what you mean?

Mathieu: Well, it's because he has a spinal cord injury and is very much into sort of staying in bed and ... it feels more like you're kind of nursing him.

Mathieu uses the phrase "take care of" intentionally, as the work he does for the client is very different from what he does for self-managers under Direct Funding. Care for Mathieu is about helping someone stay in bed rather than participate in life. As we see in the next chapter, for Mathieu, care is done by professionals, often for sick people, and is not what attendants do under Direct Funding.

Gordon, a parent advocate, confirms the connection to illness in his description of care:

People that are sick and dying may need care. And if you get really sick and have to go to the hospital you need care. But you don't need care day to day … It's the things we do to give [my son] a meaningful day! … And that's different than "care" because care assumes a debilitating thing. If I break both my legs, I need care because there are certain things I probably won't be able to do without assistance because I've injured myself.

Gordon's adult son does not have a physical impairment but an intellectual disability and is therefore ineligible for the Direct Funding Program. Gordon's comments are distanced from the Independent Living framework and suggest that other disability advocates do not want to claim care either. His definition implies that care is not enough to provide an adequate life for his son. For Gordon, care is physical, hands-on support for an individual who is debilitated, though perhaps acute support rather than ongoing. Ironically, the need for physical, hands-on support is an eligibility requirement for the Direct Funding Program and positioned as "not care" in the definition of attendant services posted on the Centre for Independent Living in Toronto's website:

Attendant Services are consumer-directed physical assistance with routine activities of daily living which the person with a disability would do him/ herself were it not for physical limitations. This assistance is provided by another person, an attendant. The consumer takes responsibility for the decisions and training involved in his/her own assistance.

Attendant Services do NOT include: professional services such as nursing care, physiotherapy, occupational therapy or physician services; respite care; supervision; "care" or taking responsibility for the person with a disability. (CILT 2000, emphasis in original)

In this definition there is no indication of the interpersonal relational work involved in attendant services, which is nevertheless mandatory for the job. Gordon's idea of care as physical assistance (albeit after an injury) starkly contrasts the Independent Living definition, which uses similar parameters to describe what care is *not*. Even though the sense of what care *is* varies in these examples, it is consistently expressed that care is not what happens here. Care is too much, and not enough, to describe the supports needed for people with disabilities. Care is for "them," over there, and this notion is even expressed by people who are implicitly and at times explicitly excluded by program eligibility requirements. As many feminist scholars argue about care work more broadly, care is devalued and likely gendered in these examples.

"Arms and Legs": Attendants as Assistive Devices

No one seems to want to be cared for, or to claim care, particularly those associated with Direct Funding. If it is not care, then what is happening in Direct Funding arrangements? For some, there is a lack of language for it, as evidenced by stammering descriptions; others speak explicitly about the ineffable nature of attendant services, such as Marie, a self-manager and Independent Living employee:

> [Attendant services are] totally, completely misunderstood. The only groups that really understand it, there's exceptions of course, are people with disabilities who use attendant services, or people who are working as an attendant. Those are the two, but I can't tell you the number of times that my attendants have said to me that they've tried to explain to their friends what they do for a living and their friends invariably don't understand.

The ambiguity of what attendant services are, aside from "not care," is reflected in the tension between two of the most dominant descriptions of attendant work: the characterization of attendants as the "arms and legs" of the self-managers, and the characterization of attendant work as a complex, interpersonal relationship. The descriptions are fluid and often both come up in the same interview, so it is not the case that certain self-managers have an "arms and legs" approach to their attendants while others have an interpersonal approach.

The "arms and legs" characterization draws on descriptions of attendant services that can be found in material produced by Independent Living organizations. For example, in CILT's publication *Powershift*, the authors note, "To understand the importance of attendants to us, think of them as our 'arms and legs'" (Parker et al. 2000, 1). As "arms and legs," attendants become extensions of the self-managers' bodies, present to pick up where the body leaves off under the direction of the self-manager, as explained on CILT's webpage (cited above). The focus is on the tasks of attendant services but, in contrast to feminist notions of caring for, this focus includes clear and firm parameters about who is responsible for determining how and when these tasks are completed (i.e., the self-manager). Self-managers are presumed to be consenting adults with physical needs, capable of self-directing their "arms and legs."

The instrumental sense that attendants are "arms and legs" is reflected by numerous participants, perhaps suggesting a thorough endorsement of the approach. Rob, an attendant, comments:

So you can almost reduce it down, I don't want to reduce it too much, but you can reduce it down to, like if I'm a little taller than you are and we're both in the kitchen and you want the rice off the top shelf, I'll just hand it to you.

Similarly, Joel, an Independent Living employee, explains:

I think the relationship, regardless of whether it's Direct Funding or Attendant Outreach – if you've got someone coming into your home to provide attendant services, they should just be an extension of your arms and legs, it should be your home and your environment and you should be able to maintain control and dignity.

The attendants are not represented as "hearts" or even "heads," which might convey a sense of charity in the first case, or professional expertise in the latter, and in both cases, arguably, more of a sense of care. Attendants are specifically "arms and legs" – disembodied, genderless, nonselves present to provide tangible assistance with specific tasks and not to offer advice or empathy, or to exercise control over the self-manager's life. In many ways, attendants are assistive devices, like a prosthetic limb, wheelchair, or Hoyer lift, operated by the directions of the self-manager. The "arms and legs" characterization contrasts the layered interpersonal descriptions to be explored shortly, descriptions indicating that not only are the whole, embodied selves of attendants required for attendant work, but that in fact uniquely combined selves are developed through relational ontologies.

Direction, Responsibility, and Automation

A substantial aspect of attendant work is following the directions of the self-managers. As "arms and legs," the attendants do not resent following directions, as they do not want to make personal, minute decisions or assume liability for someone else – and, of course, the self-managers largely agree with this approach. For example, Carolyn explains her work history as an attendant:

Yes, I worked in two different nursing homes. Yeah, and it was always different people and I did not like that ... You know, without looking at a chart, you don't know if they can eat by themselves or if they can chew or swallow or ... I don't know, just weird ... Again, I didn't like not knowing what they wanted or needed because they weren't able to tell me.

Carolyn likes that the self-managers can tell her what they want and need because this means she will not have to make assumptions or take responsibility for erroneous assumptions. She also likes the time and space Direct Funding provides to develop relationships and learn the specific needs and preferences of individual self-managers. Unfortunately, intellectual disability can become a counterpoint in helping attendants articulate what they specifically like about working under Direct Funding. Melissa, another attendant, explains:

> Well, the whole thing with a mental disability is a lot of them can't tell you what they need, right? Whereas, with just a physical disability, they can tell you what they need, so it's more, it's more of a direction, right, for Direct Funding. They tell you what you need to do.

No guessing is involved when the self-manager can articulate his or her needs to the attendant. A third example from attendant Margot:

> The boy I worked with, he was about twelve, and it was more challenging because I was more in control, right? I was supposed to be kinda telling him what to do, as opposed to being told what to do [as what happens with self-managers].

Margot does not have to tell a self-manager what to do, or figure out what he or she needs. Further, Margot does not want to be in control of the self-manager, thus resisting the domineering connotations of care. In some ways, attendants appreciate being "arms and legs" when it comes to tasks and not feeling responsible for decisions that are made while working, an appreciation that can come at the expense of people with intellectual disabilities.

The "arms and legs" characterization of attendant work in combination with the home setting creates a low-stress work environment and the recurring sense that it is "not like work," perhaps explaining why there are limited demands from attendants to improve the material working conditions. Responsibility is layered for attendants, as outside the home/work environment there is a heightened sense of obligation that goes beyond that of other types of work. Attendants are aware of how important their work is, and self-managers stress the urgency. For example, not showing up for a shift is a common reason for a self-manager to fire an attendant:

> Greg: In twelve years, I think we've fired two people. And that was for not showing up.

CK: They just didn't show up at all? Did you fire them right away or did they have a warning, or how do you normally do that?

Greg: I think they had one warning. We put up with a lot. But if you don't show up, then that, we take that seriously.

Unlike many other jobs at a similar pay, deciding not to go into work one day has profound physical and psychological consequences for the self-managers, especially for self-managers who live alone. The attendants also feel this sense of urgency. An attendant, Margot, explains:

That would probably be the one complaint about the job that I do have – is that it's very difficult if I get sick. I have had to work through a lot of shifts when I was really sick because you can't get people to come just at the last minute. No matter what, [self-managers] need someone there, right? Because otherwise they can't get up, they can't eat, they can't go to the washroom, you know? They need someone there. So I all of a sudden get sick an hour before my shift, then chances are, I'm not going get anyone to cover it, right? So I have to go in anyways.

Feeling obligated to go to work in spite of other factors is common. Hailey, an attendant, concurs:

Hailey: If you're scheduled, you have to go, and there's no one else. So, I think one time there was a ridiculous snow storm and it was my shift ... I had to walk for two hours in snow up to my waist to get to [the self-manager].

CK: Wow.

Hailey: And I had to do it, right? I mean, I couldn't leave him.

The sense of urgency and responsibility stressed by the self-managers and felt by the attendants is compounded by the sometimes rewarding but always complex relationships that the self-managers and attendants form and which reinforce feelings of obligation. However, within the home, the attendants' sense of urgency and responsibility relax. An attendant, Sheila, notes:

I think that we just work together, and it's like ... I don't know, I just find it goes so smoothly and so effortlessly. And we just know or, I guess we both know exactly what we need to do. I guess once you work with someone for quite a long time, you get to that point where it's like you just know what that person needs or know what that person wants, and I kind of like that a lot.

That is, attendants do not need to be directed step by step; rather, their actions become automatic. The self-manager's direction is working when attendants do tasks in a suitable manner without being requested to. The way tasks are "automatically" carried out is slightly (or perhaps even substantially) variable by attendant. As another self-manager describes:

> She's been assisting me for so long now that, in the mornings, it's sort of like, it's like a machine almost. It's like you know, bang, bang, bang. Or doing this, and I'm doing that, and I'm doing this, and she's maybe doing some meal prep, or something like that ... It functions very smoothly and stuff like that.

Automation in this instance does not mean thoughtless and careless actions but a comfortable deference to the self-manager in a respectful relationship similar to what might take place with a supervisor in a more traditional work environment.

Care literature exploring the use of technology in health settings suggests that technology is an impediment to relational, hands-on caring, where care is understood as a combination of physical assistance, emotional empathy, and compassion. Robots are in fact used for home care purposes but found lacking because of the missing relational components (Parks 2010; Folbre 2006). It is presumed that the emotional aspect of care "gets eaten up by technology" (Mol 2006, 5), though recent research challenges this view (Roberts, Mort, and Milligan 2012). Mol (2006, 5) critically implores, "Is care *other* to technology?"[1] and Independent Living attendants help demonstrate that it is not. In Independent Living models of support, particularly in the abstract, attendants can be interpreted as a form of assistive technology. More concretely, while working attendants utilize low-tech items such as rubber gloves, as well as high-tech devices, such as Hoyer lifts and Bliss boards. These devices operate under the direction of the self-manager in order to facilitate their daily activities. As the attendants and self-managers develop ways of being together, the actions of the attendants become automatic and do not always require direction from the self-manager. Although their actions may become automatic, attendants are not merely assistive devices; they also draw on emotional and relational skills. Curiously, even while describing attendant work in automated "arms and legs" terms, some attendants, including Carolyn, are offended by their work being reduced to mere technical actions:

---

[1] Emphasis in original.

[My friend] introduced me to her friend and he [asked] "What do you do for a living?" and my friend was kind of like, "Oh, she showers people and wipes bums and things" ... It's just funny because [of] the misconception ... You know they don't realize this person is independent. This person goes to work ... They don't see all of that and the relationship that you have.

Attendants do in fact shower people and wipe bums, but they see this work as having broader significance, stemming partially from their relationship with the self-manager and partially from the Independent Living emphasis on following self-managers' instructions. Attendants see themselves as facilitating the inclusion and participation of people with disabilities in society. Attendants are not actually assistive devices, and many features of attendant work cannot be automated, even in a metaphoric sense, namely the mandatory relational work.

Mandatory Relational Labour, Optional Friendships

The automated "arms and legs" tasks are only one component of attendant services, but many use it as a reference point to distinguish personal assistance from other forms of care. In practice, the "arms and legs" sense of Direct Funding has more to do with responsibility for decision making in daily interactions than with responsibility for the actions performed or, as feminist care scholars would highlight, a devaluing of women and gendered forms of work. Attendants, self-managers, and key informants did not want to talk much about "arms and legs" tasks. George, a former Ontario government employee during the establishment of the Direct Funding Program, summarizes the transition from "arms and legs" to more relational descriptions:

It's based on the original concept, which has been reworked now, that it's an extension of "arms and legs" for a person ... That's been modified, of course. It's been modified in part in relation to relational care, because you can only do that so much. If there's an individual, a human being, you've got to treat them that way, or all you're going to get is "arms and legs."

However, it is the combination of accepting the "arms and legs" role and the relational work that makes for good attendant services. Julie, a self-manager, stresses that attendant work is not *only* about relationships and does require a degree of technical skill:

Julie: I remember my first ever attendant, they somehow got this crazy idea in their head, the attendant, and the people who sent the attendant, that I needed a friend. So they sent someone with no attendant skills at all. And the first time she tried to use my ceiling lift, I fell out the side of the sling.

CK: Nice friend, geez!

Julie: So I said, after a couple months of that, I sat down with everyone, and I said, "I can make my own friends, thank you. I need someone to do attendant care."

Julie does not need to hire friends; she needs attendants to be her "arms and legs" first and foremost, and a friendship may or may not develop during the course of their interactions.

Martha, a parent advocate of Mark, a person with physical and intellectual disabilities (unfortunately, he had passed away by the time of the interview), eloquently describes the aspects of support that go beyond "arms and legs" in her recollection of a birthday celebration:

[The attendant] has a picture from that lunch, and I believe it's the one where she's pulling the dirty dishes out of the [shot], so it's to make it a nice picture of Mark and his sister at her birthday without it looking like he needed care, which is the ultimate, I think, in supporting somebody. To make that look seamless. To make that look like this is Mark, this is his life. My job is to clean up the dirty dishes if that makes the picture better. Whatever it takes. So calling it "care" is too narrow. It's whatever support it takes. And introducing him to the world as a person who's more than about needing care. About the contributions he could make.

Care is not enough; it is "too narrow." There is a sense that support encompasses but is more than automatically cleaning up the dirty dishes. It is not easy to describe precisely and succinctly what the "more" is that "makes the picture better." Martha alludes to relational work that attendants can do in order to highlight "the contributions" Mark and other disabled people can make, and this relational work is not considered care. It is noteworthy that Martha articulated this point of view, as her son was not eligible for Direct Funding, further indicating that it is not solely an Independent Living rejection of care.

Just as the basic technical "arms and legs" skills are, the intricate, relational side of personal support is also a necessary component of attendant work. The relational space is where the figure of the frien-tendant, to whom I can relate, sometimes emerges. Not fully employee, nor friend, nor family member, nor stranger, the frien-tendant is certainly ambiguous: extremely intimate yet also professional. It is difficult to describe these relationships, as one self-manager articulates:

> *CK:* Would you say you become friends with your other attendants?
> *Jason:* Oh yeah, definitely. Definitely – more than friends. And "friends" isn't the right word. The correlation I have to make, and this is probably a terrible correlation and if I made it in front of the people who run Self-Directed Funding, they'd probably freak out and might revoke all my funding, but it's a lot like dating. It really is. It's deeper than friendship. It's not quite dating, you know, I'm not gonna take them out on the anniversary for our first shift or anything like that. But, there is a very, very deep connection that forms, on both sides.

Comparing attendant relationships to "not-quite" dating implies a deep and ineffable intimacy. In a poem to her personal assistants, author Connie Panzarino (1996) evokes Jason's characterization by asking, "Not-a-lover-not-a-friend, but who?" Jason, among others, recounted difficulties that can arise when hiring friends or when attendants get too close: although highly intimate relationships form, their value is limited.

The relational side of attendant services is not optional: all attendants and self-managers described this aspect of work. One attendant, Rob, describes a "professional sort of closeness," likening the relationship to being cousins, whereas attendant Adam explains, "It's such intimate care that it's really impossible to keep that [employee-employer] line." The work is complicated when children, partners of self-managers, and other family members are present or involved in attendant interactions, and even more so when such people also require support from the attendant, a situation that came to light in a few interviews. This is also the space where gender, age, racialization, and other demarcations of social location are highly salient. For example, all the female self-managers in the study expressed a degree of discomfort with the idea of male attendants assisting them, particularly with intimate needs. The ineffable attendant relationship becomes too difficult to negotiate when the power dynamics shift in one direction. Compounding power differentials between disabled and nondisabled with issues of gender and sexuality in ways that make the self-manager more vulnerable when it comes to intimate "arms and legs" tasks further complicates already complicated relational work to a point where many choose to avoid hiring certain people. With the heightened vulnerability implied by estimated power imbalances (estimated, as such factors can never be measured) comes an increased risk, or perception of risk, of abuse.

The mandatory relational component of attendant services does not necessarily mean friendship; rather, it resides in the hyphen between friend and attendant. That is, although relational negotiation is always required (on the part of both attendants and self-managers), this does not invariably translate into close friendships. Two extreme examples from self-managers demonstrate this variance. When reminiscing about enjoyable times with attendants, Ryan, a self-manager, states: "So Direct Funding can be a great place to develop friendships. Like a fantastic place to make friends." Another long-term self-manager, Marc, facetiously takes an opposing view:

> I've got a rule that we don't necessarily get on [on a] friendly basis. It's fine if one day we go for a beer, but you're not going to become my best buddy, and you're not gonna ... we're not gonna have sleepovers [slight laugh], we're not gonna watch TV until the wee hours of the morning [slight laugh].

Both of these self-managers talk about how their attendants share a lot of personal information with them in conversations, and many self-managers report being sensitive to the attendants' moods (and vice versa) during the course of Direct Funding interactions. Again, in spite of the emotional connotations, this relational work is seen as "not care." It is also "not empathy": when attendants were asked if they ever required personal support or ever thought about what it would be like, most did not have much to say or seemed to avoid entertaining the thought.

As Julie explained, relationships are an important part of attendant work, but they are not the only aspect, and there is a limit to their value. Participants talked about when boundaries become too blurred and when friendships go too far. The limit to the relational side of attendant services emphasizes the sense of work that requires monitoring and thoughtfulness, particularly from the self-manager. For example, self-manager Hélène explains why she had to let a long-term attendant go:

> When you have [an attendant] for more than five years, ... they become more ... your friend, and you don't want a friend to be doing it all the time, you want someone who understands you but not someone who tells you what to do.

In a way, this self-manager is describing a time when the attendant is no longer adhering to the "arms and legs" role but too strongly asserts control and provides an unwelcome form of care. Mathieu, an attendant, echoes this sentiment, explaining the concrete implications of being too close:

> Because you pal around and joke around with that person ... There'll be effort involved, but the work kind of starts to take a hit. And you don't think that you should have to do all that much for that person because, you know ... come on, they're your buddy! Why are you asking [me] to get up and go do this, get up and go do that?

As attendants increasingly relate to the self-managers as friends, they may come to expect to interact as they do with other friends, and no longer with the unique requirements of attendant work. Elsa, another attendant, describes the emotional toll of being too close: "I wouldn't say we're 'friends *friends*,' because I think at the beginning I got a little bit too involved, and I found that that was draining me." The relationships cannot be described as light, easy friendships; they require ongoing negotiation to prevent them from veering into uncomfortable territories.

Relational Work and Emotional Labour

Despite being rewarding at times, relational negotiations are still a form of work, requiring effort and commitment by both parties. Sara expresses the sense of being "on" all the time when the attendants are in her home:

> But then on their days off sometimes, I come home and I'm like, phew! [laugh] I don't have to be cheerful! ... Someone said to me, actually, [another self-manager] said to me that he was "on" all the time. And I didn't really think about it 'til he said that. But especially for someone in his position where from the moment he wakes up to the moment he goes to bed, there's someone around. You know, I could really see that. And there is that same feeling for me [to] a lesser degree.

Here, Sara reflects the sense of managing one's emotions, as described by the concept of emotional labour originally articulated in Hochschild's study on flight attendants (1983) and in more recent developments of the concept (Wharton 2009; Steinberg and Figart 1999). In brief, emotional labour refers to the process whereby workers "induce or suppress feeling in order to sustain the outward countenance that produces the proper state of mind in others" (Hochschild 1983, 7). According to the early formulations, emotional labour is a skill required by many feminized jobs, where the workers often have to feign and sometimes deeply internalize emotions and behaviours such as cheerfulness, enthusiasm, empathy, and flirtation in order to cultivate certain moods in the clients. That is, in the service industry, the proper state of mind is the product. Yet, something distinctive is going on in Direct Funding: it is the *self-manager* who is doing the emotional management and not being paid to do it. Further, Twigg (2000) found in her study on community care and bathing that, unlike the flight attendants in Hochschild's study, attendants and some self-managers describe relational aspects as rewarding and not as a taxing part of their work (see also Korczynski 2008). Wharton (2009, 154), in her review of the concept of emotional labour within sociology, notes: "Research on caring occupations, such as nursing or midwifery, shows how change in the structure, practice and professional norms guiding these fields have the potential to increase or diminish workers' positive experience of caregiving." This is certainly the case with the Direct Funding Program, and one might argue that the potential "burden" of emotional management is diminished in the unregulated home environment of Direct Funding, where the expectations of affect are fluid or negotiated between the recipient and care worker more so than in other, more formalized care arrangements (Lopez 2006).

Payne (2009, 357) critiques the tendency to frame emotional labour as a complex skill, pointing towards individuals working in fast-food and retail industries. He argues that emotional labour is not necessarily complex, specifically when it draws on common socialization and a "basic requirement for politeness" in service work. Payne makes distinctions between "the ability to empathize" as a care worker and common manners required by other service workers, but suggests this ability is better framed as an aspect of a person's moral and ethical self. I agree with aspects of Payne's critique, particularly regarding the level of "skill" in emotional labour used in certain service jobs and the need to differentiate levels of skill in varied forms of emotional work; however, the relational work required (by both recipients and providers) in attendant services and other long-term care *is* skilled and should not be framed as a moral imperative. It is complex in that it does not draw on common socialization; it is uncommon to have, or to be, a semi-stranger involved in the intimate details of another person's life or to help an adult, or be assisted as an adult, with highly personal tasks such as bathing and toileting. No common socialization processes prepare us to carry on a "polite" conversation during these times.

In this study, self-managers talk about helping attendants become accustomed to these interactions, whereas attendants often report (and laugh about) awkward stories of their first time helping someone in the shower or toileting. For example, attendant Carolyn comments:

> At first you're showering a man and you think it's super-strange 'cause I'm just some girl off the street and I never even did nursing and I'm showering a man. But then [laugh], but then you develop a relationship and it's like, well, I don't really care who I'm showering. It's the same people that I'm always with, and it doesn't bother me at all.

The awkwardness dissipates over time as attendants learn the skills of relational work under the guidance of the self-managers, including attempting to address the power imbalances in their interactions. Furthermore, framing care work as a moral imperative undermines the hard-won rights of disability movements, placing attendant services back into the realm of charity. Carolyn further implies an aspect of the skilled relational work involved in attendant services when she says:

> A lot of times, staff don't really know how to deal with that [relational work], and if they're in a bad mood 'cause of something happened at home, they come in and they're grouchy and they're trying to hurry up ... and the client feels awkward. I'm a straight-up person. I walk in, I say, "Me and my boyfriend are having a fight. I'm in a terrible mood and it's nothing you did and I'm gonna try my best to be happy. We're gonna do this call anyway, and it's nothing you did."

Carolyn must anticipate the self-manager's reactions while evaluating and trying to control her own emotions. The self-manager on the other end of this interaction and "straight-up" announcement may be sensitive to the attendant's mood and must determine how to respond to it while being assisted with daily tasks.

The relational work is skilled, but it is not necessarily emotional labour, since it is about not only managing one's own emotions to produce a state of mind in others but also managing an ongoing relationship. Furthermore, the emotional management aspects of the job do not seem to include either the surface or deep acting aspects of emotional labour (Grandey 2003; Hochschild 1983). There is a sense of genuineness under Direct Funding that is lacking in other work environments requiring emotional labour. For example, for a young attendant named Katharine, the difference between working as an attendant and working in retail is that, in retail jobs, "you smile and nod." Self-manager Marc notes, "People that I have a better rapport [with or] whatever, they end up respecting me and they kind of end up seeing that this is for real and we're not just flipping burgers here." In some ways, attendants feel more like themselves when interacting with a self-manager than they do when working in other jobs, highlighting that doing care work is often regarded as part of one's identity (Christensen 2010; Macdonald and Merrill 2008; Cushing and Lewis 2002). Feeling genuine removes the acting but not the skill involved in emotional labour, particularly during the most intimate interactions where attendants and self-managers must learn and hone the skill of relational work.

Attendant work is too informal, relational, and personal to be framed by emotional labour. Hailey, an attendant, describes a conflict between her and the self-manager:

Hailey: I remember telling him to go fuck himself.
CK: You telling *him*?
Hailey: Yes. [After] him [having spit] water at me.
CK: Like ... not being funny, [but you were] really mad at each other?
Hailey: Yes [slight laugh]. And we still go on trips together. I don't remember what it was about, and I was so mad at him for something. And then with him, [another self-manager] will drink from the straw no matter what, but [this self-manager] will try to drink from a glass at times because it's easier. And I couldn't get it and I kept spilling water on him. And it's totally by accident. So he got mad at me and he took the water that was in his mouth and he spit it at me. And he's like, "How does it feel?" But the difference is I'm not trying to get you wet.
...
CK: What's a deal-breaker for you? ... Would you ever quit? [The self-manager] spitting water at you is ... I mean that's abusive in a way. I know we were laughing about it.
Hailey: It was more entertaining than anything because I was seriously, you just did that? [slight laugh]
CK: You have a good attitude. I would have been like "I can't believe you!" I would have freaked out.
Hailey: Yeah. But I remember [that] after I swore, because I was so mad at him. It was like "fuck this" [slight laugh]. He was like, "Let's talk about this." And he totally defused the situation ... I remember being so mad at him, I swore. And I swear, but I won't often swear at people [slight laugh].

This type of conflict sounds more like a personal argument with a family member, life partner, or close friend than it does a work-related dispute, particularly the fashion in which it was defused. Being permitted to lash out (on both sides – the self-manager's initial overreaction to the spilled water and the attendant's response) without it marking a termination of employment further indicates that the relational work required in attendant services cannot be considered emotional labour. Attendants are not required to simply smile and nod in spite of inappropriate actions of the self-managers, or vice versa, as the flight attendants are in Hochschild's study. There is more room for people to employ what attendants and self-managers regard as genuine styles of interpersonal relating within Direct Funding arrangements than there is in other service-oriented jobs where workers must pretend to care and sometimes follow preset social scripts, for example, in the case of overseas call centres (Ritzer and Lair 2008). This allowance may be directly linked to the home environment where most attendant work takes place. In emotional labour terms, attendants *and* self-managers (who are also "working" during attendant interactions) do not necessarily have to engage in surface acting and perhaps not even in deep acting, as their countenance may reflect how they truly feel at any given minute. At the same time, they must constantly interact in private spaces and moments, developing an uncommon skill set. In Direct Funding, it is about managing not only emotional reactions but a joint relationship as well.

Direct Funding interactions are a combination of mandatory, skilled, relational negotiation and accepting the role of "arms and legs" or an assistive device. Care does not encompass enough to describe the complexity of the two-way relational work, and yet it encompasses too much to describe the tasks. Philosophically, these two descriptions simultaneously reinforce and break down distinctions between the autonomous self and interdependently intertwined selves. Disembodied arms fill in the gaps of bodies with disabilities, correcting what Garland-Thomson (2011) terms "misfits" and maintaining a semblance of the myth of autonomy. But attendants are not body parts; the physicality, intimacy, and isolation of attendant work under Direct Funding demand and create new ways of relating and interpreting the boundaries of the self.

Chameleon Attendants and Responsive Self-Managers

The tension between the "arms and legs" descriptions of attendant services that abound in Independent Living perspectives and the mandatory, complex relational work in which no assistive device can be directed is not entirely unexpected, as suggested by a few other studies and my own observations before this study (e.g., Gibson et al. 2009; Hughes et al. 2005; Earle 1999). Attendants and self-managers manage this ambiguity by developing relational strategies. For attendants, particularly those who do attendant work with more than one person, this often means adopting a chameleon-like personality. Mathieu describes the work required to relate with a variety of people:

> *Mathieu:* I'm not like a chameleon, but I can sort of still be myself. Yet, I've always sort of been able to kind of, my personality has rarely really clashed with a lot of people for the most part because when I'm thinking of it, I can always sort of try to adapt ... I guess it's kind of [a] personality that I can kind of switch over and kind of adapt and tune into somebody else's personality and meet them at that place ...
>
> *CK:* So, would they sort of take the lead a bit?
>
> *Mathieu:* They take the lead a little bit, and I'll sort of work from there and find out a little more about them and try to sort of connect with them after they've taken the lead ...
>
> *CK:* Find something you connect on.
>
> *Mathieu:* And yeah, and then we have a bit of a common thing going on and I don't walk into a room and say, "Here's me!"
>
> *CK:* I'm here!
>
> *Mathieu:* "Here's my personality, this is what I'm all about! And ... what are you, not like me? I just kind of try to sort of sit in the shadows for a bit and see what's happening and what people are all about.

The attendants who do this work for the longest seem to embody this type of flexibility, perhaps reflecting Waerness's rationality of caring (1996). Experienced attendants can work just as easily with a formal employer style of one self-manager as they can with an informal, relaxed style of another. Attendants are present beyond following directions and doing tasks, responding relationally to the self-managers.

Feminist studies on care often focus on the efforts of care workers, yet this relational work is two-way (Marfisi 2010). Many of the self-managers expressed that they were being responsive to their attendants by taking into account their gender, age, and social position. For example, self-manager Ryan explained that when he goes on vacation, he is aware of the impact it will have on his attendants, who will not be paid during his absence. He is particularly concerned about his attendants who are attending university or college and tries to give them extra shifts leading up to his time away, "because the young ones always worry about money." That is, self-managers acknowledge that not all "arms and legs" are the same. Self-managers develop incredibly empathetic interpersonal skills that in part shield against abuse and the legacies of institutionalization, as both recipients and attendants are humanized. Self-managers talk about being easygoing with attendants, and despite the emphasis on consumer direction, self-managers leave room for attendants to express their own interests and ideas, and even to perform attendant tasks in their own ways. The Independent Living emphasis on consumer direction wavers as attendants participate in decision making, complete specific tasks in their own ways, and develop elements of "automation" when they no longer require step-by-step instructions. Long-term attendant Hailey recounts a clear example of a responsive self-manager:

> *Hailey:* With [one self-manager] I found out he would rather finish one
> whole thing. Like on his meal, on a plate, say your potatoes, meat, and
> carrots. He'd rather finish all of his carrots and then all of his meat, then
> all of his potatoes, [rather] than picking and choosing bits and pieces of
> it. It wasn't even [the self-manager] that told me this. It was somebody,
> I think it was [his friend] that was upstairs at dinner one night. And
> she looks at me and looks at [the self-manager] and she goes, "I thought
> you liked your meal this way?" And he's like, "Well, I do." I'm like, "Shit!
> I've been working for you like two years, why haven't you said anything?"
> *CK:* You didn't tell me, yeah?
> *Hailey:* He's like, "Well, it's not really that big of a deal."

Hailey was surprised that the self-manager does not mind how he is assisted during meals; she had assumed she was being his "arms and legs" and following his directions, letting him take the lead.

Beyond making room for attendants to develop their own ways of doing certain tasks, all the self-managers described being a sympathetic ear for their attendants, often as a strategy for helping new attendants feel at ease, particularly during intimate tasks. For example, self-manager Marc notes, "Yeah, I become the, I don't know, the psychologist of the place. 'My boyfriend this!' It's like, ah-ha! Here we go again!" Margot, a young attendant, recounts how the self-manager she works for is sensitive to her social anxiety:

> We're so open, especially [the self-manager I work for] knows me really
> [well] now. For example, I have a lot of social anxiety so big crowds, going
> to the mall, sometimes creates anxiety. And [the self-manager] will actually

ask me now because she knows me. "Are you okay with this? Does this make you anxious? Let me know if you get feeling anxious," you know?

Self-managers are active recipients of support in multiple ways, from subtle physical accommodations to relational management. Give-and-take with attendants is seen as a significant part of being a self-manager and creating a positive working environment. Shauna, an advocate and self-manager, describes the importance of give-and-take:

> One of the advantages with Direct Funding is the direct accountability between you and your worker, which leads to much more respect and support for each other. For example, if a worker said to you, "My kid, the school pageant is tonight, and it's going to make me really late getting to you." Then I would say, "Oh heck, I don't mind! Even if you come at midnight, that's okay." In turn, maybe I want to go out one night and won't [need help going to bed] 'til midnight, and [so] talk to the worker about it and say, "You know, I'd really like to go to this." And the worker would say, "Oh yeah, sure." It's a give-and-take.

Give-and-take and having an empathetic ear are important, as self-managers want to make sure attendants feel appreciated and will want to stay for extended periods. Self-manager Cheryl describes it this way:

> And that's why I try to get to know them [on a] personal basis. You know, and try to be interested in each one. And then try to remember what they said [slight laugh]. Try not to make it all about me, you know? Because that's what it is, it's all about me.

The ambiguity between distanced "arms and legs" that follow directions and advanced interpersonal skills is generally managed by adopting chameleon and responsive approaches. Yet, these approaches are actually quite similar, blurring the distinction between attendant and self-manager roles and intentions. Ironically, the attendants talk about being chameleons by "sitting in the shadows," as Mathieu says, in order to let the self-managers take the lead, whereas the self-managers use empathy and relax their expectations of how certain tasks should be completed in order to make room for the varied social locations and personalities of their attendants. Neither is truly happening, then; the attendants are not overshadowing, nor are the self-managers shining and completely directing the interactions. Attendants and self-managers interact in a space where new forms of relating are created by attempting to bend to one another. Fritsch (2010, 11) draws on Deleuze and Guattari to theorize these moments as "relational assemblages," arguing: "The emphasis, then, is placed not on what you can do for me but rather what we can create together." Gibson (2006, 192) draws on the same theorists and describes an attendant facilitating sexual interactions for people with disabilities:

> The attendant is expected to be a detached "tool" for facilitating their coupling – a means to an end. Despite knowing her role, she experiences a leaking of her identity, a mingling of her own sexuality with theirs; their coupling is also hers (a ménage).

Assistance with sexual interactions stretches and challenges the common definitions of "intimate," but a blurring of identities in attendant relationships occurs beyond those types of activities. Erickson (2007, 45), a self-proclaimed queer femmegimp, describes her personal support:

> The care that I need requires a lot of physical and intimate touch and contact, not to mention coordination. References to dancing occur on many occasions as my personal assistants help me because of the constant conscious and unconscious negotiation that has to transpire between us. This negotiation occurs because my personal assistant and I, and our bodies, are functioning as a self and as a unit.

Leading and following, asserting personality, advising, directing, and doing blend together. Unlike many of the participants in this study, Fritsch, Gibson, and Erickson are not wary of care; they embrace the messiness, blurred boundaries, and mashing of identities implied by care in their descriptions (see also Hamington 2004; Price and Shildrick 2002). Arguably, the participants in this study do so as well, though implicitly at the point where chameleon and responsive strategies merge into a unified approach, or dance, as Erickson describes. In a poem dedicated to her "other bodies," Panzarino (1996, 85) articulates the relational ontology of attendant work:

> *I spend more time with you than with my lover.*
> *Our boundaries blur with painful necessity*
> *as I know when you are hungry, but saying you're not,*

or constipated, or doubting yourself,
and you suffer my medical abuses as if they were your own,
Just as you know my everything
from my love of chocolate, my bank balance, and what
brand of tuna I buy
to how my twisted body must be placed at night so
that we both get a good night's sleep.

Panzarino and her attendant operate both as a self and as a unit, concerned about each other's physical dis/comfort in order to protect their own. In another piece of poetry, Stacey Milbern (2009), also known as cripchick, offers a sexually charged description of getting dressed, revealing she is writing about an interaction with her attendant only in the final stanza. Erickson, Panzarino, and Milbern all identify as queer women with disabilities, and Milbern adds that she is a woman of colour. These women eloquently describe the relational ontologies forged in attendant work and embody complexity. They do not reduce themselves, nor attendant work, to simple or singular definitions. The weaving, conflicting descriptions of "arms and legs," prosthetics, and complex relational work managed through mutually respectful deference deeply challenge the power imbalances and dependencies linked to care.

Closing Thoughts

Independent Living echoes strongly in the descriptions of attendant services as "not care," yet the picture painted of personal assistance also resonates with feminist descriptions of care. That is, separating the instrumental side of "caring for" from the emotional sense of "caring about" echoes the separation of task-based "arms and legs" descriptions from the ambiguous but mandatory relational work (Grant et al. 2004; Finch and Groves 1983). So then, what makes personal assistance different from care?

We cannot ignore the push away from care found in this study and in others, and this is primarily why the caring for/caring about distinction cannot be directly employed. From the descriptions in the interviews, directing or being directed to do a certain task (whether it happened at one point in time or is ongoing) – for example, putting on socks and shoes – changes the nature and experience of the task for both recipient and attendant. This is the case even if the end result is the same (i.e., you end up wearing your socks and shoes), and the experience can be accurately described only as "not care." Care encompasses too much in this situation, it has too much baggage, as Jennifer says; it is much simpler to talk about concrete tasks and stress the importance of consumer direction. The painful histories, legacies, and ongoing practices of institutionalization are too close to embrace care. For attendants, being directed instead of making decisions in the best interest of your "charge" (Kittay 1999; Wong and Millard 1992) changes the experience of performing the tasks in significant ways. In fact, the attendants expressed that they did not want the decision-making responsibility – they did not want the onus of making the "right" decision to be on them – or as Tronto (1993, 106) terms it, to assume the "taking care of" element of care. The attendants specifically like working in an Independent Living model and may not do this work within another framework. Calling attendants "arms and legs" is a reminder that the self-manager is in charge and is liable, but this does not deny the existence of a whole self, or even combined self, as revealed in the relational labour and relational ontologies developed.

In terms of the mandatory relational work, attendant services can be distinguished from other descriptions of caring about in important ways. Primarily, while a fondness for the self-managers makes personal support smoother, friendship or familial forms of relating are not required. The relational work that does take place can be much more complicated. As most clearly demonstrated by the comments of parent advocates, "care" is not enough to describe these aspects. New relational terms are established within each attendant relationship, and renegotiated through each interaction, as demonstrated by the chameleon/responsive self-manager. Attendants and self-managers may relate as friends in one instance, as employee and employer in others, and this constant shifting of roles requires skilled relational work. This work helps avoid confrontation and clashes in personality, and takes into account gender, age, and life position. Arguably, relational work is involved in care as generally understood; however, the personal assistance environment under Direct Funding highlights the role of self-managers in doing this work. This relational work is an active, two-way process that must be done by both the attendants and the people who require support, and it does not require as much acting as other service jobs; for these reasons, among others, it cannot be adequately explained by the concept of emotional labour. For the self-managers, the relational work includes making attendants feel at ease and appreciated, building rapport in order to instill a sense of responsibility when outside the work environment, and maintaining an awareness of potential forms of abuse and the legacies of institutionalization. The self-managers' relational work builds on critiques of care by asserting agency through directing their attendants, being vigilant against potentially dangerous and abusive situations, and trying to preserve a home environment that is not institutionalized.

Direct Funding is not care because the responsibility is in the hands of the self-managers, and the relational work is two-way, mandatory, and more complex than forming friendships or familial relationships. At this point, it can appear as though, just as in CILT's description of attendant services, care does not happen here. However, the resistance to care was not universally expressed through the course of the interviews: a few participants were surprised that care was rejected, and at some point almost all participants used the term "care" in a relatively neutral fashion. Many (in fact, as many as who firmly rejected care) expressed indifference towards the word on the condition that personal support is done in an Independent Living manner. There is ambivalence towards care even within this paradigm example of Independent Living, as well as a sense that care does not disappear with the advent of Direct Funding. Care still happens "out there" and "somewhere else"; occasionally, it does happen "here" within Direct Funding, as we explore in the next chapter.

4

Exploring the "Authentic Times to Care"
The Places Where Care Belongs

Independent Living movements distance themselves from care as a means to empowering disabled people, introducing new policy mechanisms for community and social service delivery, and challenging pervasive negative conceptions of disability and dependency. These are compelling strategies, many of which appear in the context of the Direct Funding Program, where the interactions between self-managers and their attendants are largely described with alternative concepts. It appears as though the Independent Living messages documented in academic literature are clearly replicated in public documents and by public figures, and more creatively interpreted within Direct Funding. In short, "We don't need care," and care does not happen within Independent Living models of support. Yet, surprisingly, care still takes place. There are times when "care" is the only possible description – for example, community activist Johanna explains:

> The authentic times to care for people are when they're born or when they're dying. You know, when they're suffering deeply in some way. It's great in its rightful place, but it locates us as children or sick or dying one way or the other.

Even though the majority of participants in this study reject the term "care" in some way, this rejection does not mean that care completely disappears. Further, very few of the participants completely abandon the term, and some imply that there are places where care belongs, as demonstrated by Johanna's statement.

Care emerges as an ambiguous and at times unwelcome set of actions and attitudes that we all have to tolerate at some points in our lives and which is necessary and even appropriate for certain people, particularly those who are sick or those who cannot self-direct.

The process of refining and containing the meanings of care complicates debates between feminist care researchers and critical disability perspectives. Containing care demonstrates that the debates should not be framed in terms of independence versus inter/dependence or in terms of care versus support. Disavowing care within Independent Living frameworks, even to the extent of removing it from public documents, does not eliminate it. This discursive move does make it difficult to see what happens to care, and thus care and independence become the distracting focal points in divergent perspectives. Moving the concept of care away from Independent Living but allowing it to remain in other areas changes the meanings of care and reduces its oppressive potentials. Before expanding on this argument, I explore four key areas that still count as care according to the participants in this study; that is, care is an intricate form of oppression; linked to medical and social professionals; a necessary set of actions during times of illness, for specialized medical treatments, and highly intimate needs; and an approach to supporting people with intellectual disabilities and others who cannot self-direct.

Care as Oppression

Just as disability studies literature argues, for some participants in this study, care is seen as a complex form of oppression that must be removed from the Direct Funding Program. There are three key aspects of this oppression: the erasure of agency for those who require support; the legacies of institutionalization; and, to cite Michael Fine's term (2007, 4), the "dark side" or potential for abuse and coercion, all of which surfaced at various points in the interviews. One of the strongest critiques of care comes from key informant Jim, a long-term disability leader who was central to establishing the program:

> Care is ... the *ersatz* model of love, in other words, like coffee made out of chicory. It's not real love and it's not real care. Care is where someone else is responsible for you. And that's the most important concept of the word "care." They care for you. And to this day, my family still thinks that these attendants care for me; the locus of control, then, is with the caregiver; the locus of responsibility is with the caregiver. And the disabled person, the object of care, becomes an invalid, or "in-valid," and has no control over

their own body functions in the sense of their own needs, or has at least limited control. And we wanted to get away from the word "care." Care is for sick people who can't help themselves. That's where it belongs properly, so it's an extraction from the medical model. That's our biggest enemy, and it always has been – the medical model – 'cause we are conceptualized by the general public as needing care.

Even in this passionate rejection of care, Jim suggests that care does not completely disappear. Jim states, "It's not real love and it's not real care," implying that there are forms of care that *are* real, and times and places where it does belong. Just as there is imitation coffee made out of chicory, there are false forms of care directed at people with disabilities. What remains to be seen, however, is what "real" care is. Ironically, "real" care – accessible care – may be in fact found in Independent Living models of support, which explicitly reject the idea of care. Or, as Cheryl, a self-manager puts it: "I guess Independent Living is what takes care of me."

Any definition of care must include an acknowledgement of its oppressive sides, including the potential for abuse and coercion of those who require support and those who provide it. Behind all the positive evaluations of Direct Funding in Canada and elsewhere (e.g., Yoshida et al. 2004; Glendinning et al. 2000; Maglajlic, Brandon, and Given 2000), there remains an ever-looming oppressive side to care. Even in this small study, participants alluded to the vulnerability of self-managers and attendants, and some directly recounted instances of crisis – financial, physical, verbal, or sexual abuse – to varying degrees of severity. The oppressive side of care is not a metaphor or abstract rallying slogan ("disabled people are oppressed by care") but a daily possibility drawing on lived experiences of vulnerability, abuse, and coercion. Although care scholars deftly point out how obligations to provide both formal and informal care unfairly implicate women (Glenn 2010), and that caregivers can be abused by recipients (Michael Fine 2007), this scholarship does not pay adequate attention to the potential and ongoing oppression of disabled people. Whether or not feminist scholars agree, these experiences are intertwined with the concept of care for many participants in this study.

In nearly every interview participants spoke of the risks of self-managers being stranded because an attendant does not show up or unexpected needs arise. This risk ranges from minor to more serious examples. On the minor end, Rita, an informal support, describes her main concern with Direct Funding: "Say for instance she's writing or typing and she drops something. And she needs it. Who's gonna pick it up?" This situation is annoying, but it is not life threatening, painful, or even uncomfortable. Those who use Direct Funding are implicitly, and sometimes explicitly, drawn to the Independent Living model that builds on deinstitutionalization. In addition to promoting living in the community in nonmedicalized environments, Independent Living presumes that the freedom to make seemingly mundane decisions is a necessary component of full inclusion. One of the most dehumanizing aspects of institutionalization is the lack of control over daily decisions and the imposition of routine (Goffman 1961). When the Direct Funding model cannot logistically account for all daily decisions (e.g., wanting to pick up something that has dropped), it is a substantive critique that references the oppressive legacies of institutionalization.

There were also accounts and concerns about more serious vulnerabilities and forms of oppression inherent in Direct Funding. Jason describes a situation dating back to when he had just started using Direct Funding:

> I'm still really fresh and new at this and [the attendant] misses her third shift. She calls me about two hours before her shift and asks if she's working tomorrow. And I'm like, "No, you work tonight!" And she's like, "Oh, because I'm [out of town], so I'm not gonna be able to get in tonight." So I freaked out, and I had no idea what to do, right? Like, this is the first time anything like this has happened, and my mom wasn't there and here was that moment of panic ... So it's that moment of, I'm not going to be able to survive. I'm not going to be able to do this. So I slept in my chair that night. I didn't sleep very much, you know, it's pretty hard to sleep in an electric wheelchair.

Ever looming with Direct Funding, given its increased flexibility and freedom, are minor and substantial vulnerabilities that can lead to experiences of discomfort, abuse, and forms of oppression, particularly for those who live alone. Other self-managers describe the importance of emergency back-up systems, as well as a sense of panic when attendants are late or do not show up. One self-manager recounted the terrible experience of an attendant missing a morning shift, forcing him to soil the bed. The unease and panic came up frequently in interviews and undergirds the experience of Direct Funding. Indeed, this side of attendant support is partly why Saxton and colleagues (2001) argue for an expanded definition of abuse that includes stranding a person with a disability.

Unfortunately, accounts of more typical forms of physical, sexual, emotional, and financial abuse also emerged in the interviews, again underlining the tangible nature of defining care as a form of oppression. These abuses were more common in attendant arrangements other than under Direct Funding. Under the latter, there were mostly examples of attendants stealing money and belongings from the self-managers. One self-manager recounts:

I had a friend who got kicked off Self-Directed Funding because he had an attendant who was abusing him and he didn't know what to do. He didn't know who to talk to or where to go. And the attendant stole a ton of money from him. A lot of it was from the self-directed fund, where she made him sign cheques for her. She would just empty out his attendant care budget basically, and he was too shy and too afraid of this woman to say anything. And so they kicked him off Self-Directed Funding when everything came unravelled. They were like, "Well, clearly you're not capable of directing your own funding because you were just taken for thousands and thousands of dollars by this woman." It's a situation where there was violence and that ... would never happen to me because I would call the cops.

Discussions of abuse took on at times a distinctly gendered tone. A female self-manager vaguely recounts an instance of abuse:

CK: Do you ever have a man as an attendant?
Self-Manager: Yes, I did. And I had to make him leave too.
CK: You had to make him leave too?
Self-Manager: He was abusing. Abusing.
CK: Oh, I'm sorry. That's terrible.
...
Self-Manager: Yeah. But he was an abuser a long time. He's been in prison for abusing.
CK: Oh god.
Self-Manager: But you don't know that.
CK: Did you report him to the police?
Self-Manager: Ah no, because they didn't ... okay what happened was [I] went to Independent Living for, to help for that, to make him go. But I didn't have any attendant. But my thinking was not all there. I was so tired emotionally and physically and all that. Like, I didn't think of anything. They were gonna bring me to a shelter for a while. But there was no shelter for disabled people available at that time.

As other researchers find (e.g., Millen 1997), it was difficult to open direct discussions about gender; however, the one exception was discussing men working as attendants for female self-managers. All the female self-managers in this study expressed some degree of concern about having male attendants. Some stated quite strongly that they hire only women, whereas others reported that they permit male attendants to assist with tasks that are not considered personal care, such as housework, help with meals, and eating. A female self-manager says: "I kind of care [about the gender of my attendants] for some things, for like going to the washroom." It was implied or directly stated that this preference was out of concern not only for modesty but also for potential abuse. For example, another female self-manager says:

> You're giving them a key to your house ... I'm not necessarily comfortable in giving some random male stranger I don't know a key to [my] home, knowing full well that if, you know, who knows what can happen. Women can [inaudible] abuse too, but chances are, we know statistics, it's gonna be a male.

Attendant–self-manager interactions include power differentials that the Independent Living approach attempts to address; that is, attendants have a form of physical power over the self-managers, and the self-managers counter this with the power associated with making decisions and acting as employers. The power differentials are precariously negotiated in and out of balance through the difficult relational work outlined in the previous chapter. These delicate differentials can be easily pushed out of balance when the attendants occupy powerful social identities, such as when an able-bodied male attendant supports a female self-manager, especially with her most intimate needs. Although the female attendants largely feel they could work with either male or female self-managers, the male attendants, with a couple of exceptions, felt varying degrees of discomfort about the idea of helping women. Attendant Mathieu:

> It's just a risky situation. Especially since you're going to be doing this [inaudible] privately in a room somewhere and this involves you taking off some vulnerable person's clothes and helping them. And anything could happen, where you feel you're helping them and that person feels that you actually touched them inappropriately. But, obviously, if you're helping them in the washroom, there might be a chance that you might touch them somewhere they wouldn't want to be touched.

There is no formula to predict when the power differentials will be more or less pronounced. It is easier for female self-managers to categorically avoid hiring men as attendants than it is to attempt to predict and negotiate these complex imbalances on an individual basis. This wholesale exclusion, which is sometimes the policy in other attendant arrangements, may offend long-term attendants, such as the one who says:

> I discussed this with one of the administrators [at another place I worked] because I thought it was sort of assuming that male attendants are going to behave badly or sexually assault the people that they're helping. And I was kind of offended by that actually, because why is it more likely for a male attendant to do that than it is for a female attendant?

As one participant noted, it is statistically more likely for a male attendant to abuse than for a female attendant to do so. The balance of power can be offset in other ways – for example, when women of colour work as care providers, they often experience forms of racism from clients of different backgrounds (Neysmith and Aronson 1997).

Under Direct Funding, self-managers are willing to take on these major and minor vulnerabilities and potential sites of oppression, gendered and otherwise, again gesturing towards the legacies of institutionalization. And those legacies of institutionalization are not a distant past. The last residential treatment centre closed in Ontario in 2009, yet similar institutions continue to operate in other provinces. The historic class-action lawsuit against the Ontario government related to abuse and mistreatment in the regional centres came forward in 2012. In a broader landscape, many long-term residential homes that operate in Ontario serve predominantly older people and, occasionally, adults with physical disabilities, and many group homes or attendant-service arrangements continue to operate with an institutionalized approach to disability. Even in this study, at least two of the participants spent a large part of their childhoods in institutions. Although self-managers (and those who support them) do not want the constant surveillance, structure, and systemic exclusion, among many other atrocities, that are associated with institutions, institutions may provide protection from specific vulnerabilities, namely being stranded. Institutions certainly do not protect from the risks of abuse and, in fact, a higher risk of abuse exists for people with disabilities in institutions than in community arrangements (Rajan 2004). This conundrum between protection and vulnerability, revealed in the accounts of being stranded and even in the brief comment about what might happen if a self-manager "drops something," demonstrates the paradoxical complexities of care: in a single instance, care can be empowering, risky, oppressive, healing, and secure.

The instances of abuse are disturbing, but the participants emphasized that experiences of this aspect of care were uncommon. However, if we are using the expanded definition of abuse proposed by Saxton and colleagues (2001) that includes being stranded, this form of abuse was very common and is a limitation of the Direct Funding Program. This type of work can be physically and emotionally demanding, with no employment benefits, particularly no sick days. The issue of attendants missing work, though a serious and important concern, also highlights problematic working conditions that accompany this model of support.

The common experience of being stranded accompanied with mild to profound anxiety becomes a harsh reminder of dependency. There are moments where the environment fails to accommodate physical differences and thus, as the social model of disability would suggest, these moments create experiences of disability (Oliver 1990). During these moments, self-managers must face the systematic oppression against people with disabilities embedded in structural environments. Isabelle, a self-manager, explains:

> *Isabelle:* We've had those kind of situations where I think there's something wrong. When the money's there, yet we can't have basic needs met because [people don't show up or we can't find new attendants to hire]. I worry about that. But not very often. It doesn't happen often, but it takes one time to think, "Wow, we are really dependent." Right?
> *CK:* You only notice when the system breaks.
> *Isabelle:* Exactly. Exactly.
> *CK:* You know it's going along fine, everything is going well, and then all of a sudden ...
> *Isabelle:* It's like the van. When my van breaks down ... I don't notice my disability until my van breaks down and I can't take the bus or [the accessible bus service], whatever, because I'm not going to get to work on time ... Um, that's when I notice, okay, I am disabled, okay? Right? Or the scooter breaks down, see, I don't notice it until my infrastructure doesn't work.

There is a profound aversion to these moments. Reminders of dependency reveal the power dynamic that Independent Living and the Direct Funding Program work so hard to subvert, and happen in reference to technology breaking down or attendants as metaphorical "assistive devices" not showing up for work. Garland-Thomson presents the idea of the misfit to advance the social model of disability. According to Garland-Thomson (2011, 593), "The discrepancy between body and world, between that which is expected and that which is, produces fits and misfits." Moments of vulnerability and dependency for self-managers highlight the "discrepancy between body and world" and represent uncomfortable reminders of an environment that presumes a mythical autonomous, able-bodied norm.

In many cases, the attendant ultimately holds a form of power over the self-manager, who is dependent on attendants in order to meet basic needs. This power contains a high potential to veer towards abuse or coercion, especially in terms of leaving someone stranded. This dynamic is sometimes disrupted for those who have trusted informal supports – a partner, spouse, child, roommate, or relative sharing the same living space – who can fill in when needed. Just as the issue of attendants not showing up is more complicated than it first appears, the aversion to reminders of physical dependency affects the attendants as well. Attendants express a high degree of responsibility outside the work environment. They often go in to work to assist the self-manager when in other types of employment they would take the day off (e.g., because of illness). Even in the most emancipatory models of support, the vulnerabilities of care do not disappear.

A few attendants reported instances of abuse, mainly verbal in nature. As feminist scholars argue, care can also be oppressive for those who provide it, whether through abusive recipients of support or more broadly through unstable working conditions and social devaluation of their skills (Kittay 1999). Attendant Andrea recounts a situation in which another attendant was sneaking around behind the self-manager:

> *Andrea:* No, I didn't say anything [about this other attendant to the self-manager] because she was so abusive it was hard.
> *CK:* Was it verbally abusive?
> *Andrea:* Yeah, that I have a horrible laugh, I wasn't allowed to talk loudly, she was gonna shoot me down, like constantly.

Other attendants spoke about abuse, but not in the first person and again outside of Direct Funding. For example, one attendant says,

> More often, I should say, as an aside to that, there [were] more incidents of attendants being put into positions where they felt uncomfortable or being propositioned [sexually] or what not. It went that way a lot more than it

ever, I mean, I didn't hear a single client who had been in any way abused by an attendant, but it did go the other way.

Another attendant says,

I guess just "abused" in that [attendants are] talked down to and there's disparaging remarks made. That same client that I was talking about earlier ... who had a conflict with me, who accused me of stealing things, he actually ended up getting ... I guess essentially kind of squeezed out of [the living arrangement] because there were just too many incidents in which he was just making too many inappropriate comments to the female staff.

Oppression, abuses, and vulnerability are a very real part of care for people in this study and in broader disability perspectives. Further, for those who reject the term "care," sometimes the oppressive sides become equated with care in its entirety and translated into "what we don't want" or "not what happens here." At times, care is seen only as oppression, but definitions are fluid and this meaning does not hold for long. There are other concepts linked to care, for example, professionalism, responsibility for health, and personal needs and support for people with intellectual disabilities. Rejecting care and its oppressive potentials does not eliminate these other elements, since there are increasing moves to professionalize and regulate workers, people with physical disabilities will have health-related needs that push the boundaries of home care, and people with intellectual disabilities also require attendant services.

Professionals and the Direct Funding Program

Independent Living movements include resistance to professionalism, since "care" professionals are seen as privileged people who presume to know what is in the best interests of a passive client. The hesitancy towards professionals remains in this study, and contrasts with (and perhaps impedes) the political galvanization to standardize developmental service workers and the proliferation of personal support worker (PSW) training programs in Canadian colleges.

According to Adams (2010), the concept of profession is difficult to define and varies across time and context. Even medicine, the "epitome of professionalism," is "intrinsically intertwined with the values of society within which doctors practice" (van Mook et al. 2009, 81 and 82). In trait-based definitions of professions, items such as training, professional associations, regulation, protection of jurisdiction, and ethics are used as criteria to determine what is considered a profession (Hwang and Powell 2009). Adams (2010) advocates for a focus on regulation as the key to identify what constitutes a profession, suggesting the significance of discussions on regulating support workers. Adams further adds the roles of status and power, which were not included in trait-based definitions until the 1980s. When groups and individuals critique the notion of professionals, such as views expressed by disability advocates, the concern seems to be with an unfounded expertise and the power to assert that point of view. There is the additional behavioural component, as some researchers explore how to teach professional*ism* in medical school (Cruess and Cruess 2006) and how to identify when medical professionals behave "unprofessionally," implying a sense of politeness and formality (Hickson et al. 2007). Resisting forms of formal professional behaviour is a manifestation of larger critiques of the power and privilege associated with professions.

Critiques of professionals emerged in this study as well. Community advocate and self-manager Shauna recalls her involvement in a consultation exploring the possibility of regulating PSWs:

> There was a marvellous woman there who was from the Older Women's Network. Anytime she would open her mouth, some of the professional people would look at her and smile and say, "Isn't she cute?" And I would say something, and the RNs and the professionals would be very whatever. [My friend], who is an RN, who is very Independent Living consumer-oriented, would say the same thing, but because she is an RN, they would listen to her.

In Shauna's account, professionals are given more respect and authority than are the self-advocates. The registered nurse may or may not identify as a disabled person, but she has an Independent Living orientation. Care professionals have the power to "speak for" people with disabilities but may or may not have the "right" perspective to do so. George, a former senior manager with the Ontario Ministry of Health and Long-Term Care, explains:

> [If the broader home care system] starts seriously thinking about a direct-funding model, which they have to someday, it [will be difficult because it's] such a medical model and in that case, the disabled community is correct. Nobody wants to give up that control. Health professionals are trained, they're risk-adverse, and they're trained to make decisions for other people in spite of the fact that they say they don't do that, that they get consent.

As other scholars (e.g., Matthias and Benjamin 2008; Caldwell and Heller 2003) find, some self-managers prefer to hire people with no attendant experience and take particular issue with those who graduate from PSW programs. This preference has a long history in Independent Living, as seen in successful efforts to exempt attendants from the Regulated Health Professions Act and the early days of Independent Living in the United States, when "disabled students initially found their workforce among other students and wartime conscientious objectors, helpers who never envisioned attendant care as a long-term occupation or on that required any special training" (Boris and Klein 2006, 107). In this study, Joel, an Independent Living employee, explains, "Yeah, we get people in [with PSW diplomas], and we have to un-train them and then train them again." This implies that attendants do require training, but not the training provided in credentialed programs that train them "to make decisions for other people." Although representatives of Independent Living often speak about attendants as "arms and legs," it is implied that these extremities are not interchangeable; the skills required to be a good attendant cannot be universally taught in a formal program.

PSWs are seen as proponents of the medical model. Medicine is the "epitome of profession" (van Mook et al. 2009, 81) and, as Jim said earlier, "That's our biggest enemy, and it always has been – the medical model." Other participants echo this sentiment in the sense of wanting to prove medical care professionals wrong. Theresa, an informal support and mother of a self-manager, reflects back on advice given to her when her son was first diagnosed:

> I don't know why [the doctors and professionals] tell you that anyway. You know, just let you deal with the news [about your infant's disability] they've given you to begin with. They don't need to tell you that your marriage isn't gonna last, and that your son should be in an institution. Yeah, but anyway, so we proved them wrong.

By proving them wrong, self-managers and their supports can reveal the limited knowledge of care professionals. Martha, a parent advocate whose son, Mark, had profound intellectual and physical disabilities, recounts her son's assessment by professionals:

> *Martha:* We applied to I think two agencies somebody told us about. They came to interview Mark to determine whether he could "direct his own care." We had been agents of that. And there'd been people who knew

him in a lot of different ways, who understood how he directed his own care with us in the picture. So, it was a really tough morning when that woman came. I was really tense. I was really sure that they were gonna say he wasn't able to direct his own care, because they wanted to interview him privately.

CK: Oh my gosh.

Martha: I was getting really tense, and Mark must have picked that up. We're all in the living room waiting for this person to come, and he turned on the most babyish cartoon show that he never ever watched. It was like *Teletubbies* or something. And he never watched that, he always watched –

CK: Adult shows?

Martha: Well, he'd watch cartoons, but they were always of the more cerebral type. And I was like, "That's really making me mad! This person is gonna assess!" I didn't wanna say anything, but I was communicating it, and he was like "Screw you, I don't care to be assessed." And my husband said, "Well, they can't interview him because they don't know sign language." So the woman came and [my husband] says, "Do you know sign language?" "Oh, no, no." "How would you interview Mark privately if you don't know sign?" – even though Mark had some other methods, but they were always interspersed with sign. So, it was like "Oh, I can't! Okay, well, you stay in the room then." So, we had a sort of interdependent assessment, and he passed.

This story is saturated with the sense of wanting to convince the professionals to get the required services, rather than seeing the assessment as fair and objective. Martha and the actions of Mark suggest that the professional assessment is unlikely to capture the creative, complex, and relational ways of directing and communicating that the family cultivated over a long period. Mark and his family, who experientially and deeply know how attendant services work in their household, are pressured to present this intangible information in an acceptable format that will result in a sufficient amount of services (for a more detailed analysis of assessment, see Kelly and Chapman 2015).

Eva Feder Kittay (2010) urges moral philosophers to express "epistemic modesty" (to know what you don't know) and "epistemic responsibility" (to know the subject for whom you claim to speak) when debating the value of the lives of people with profound disabilities; some participants in this study take this even further by implying that professionals cannot practice epistemic responsibility in relation to attendant services. This is further supported by the discussions in the previous chapter on the difficulty in describing the nature of attendant interactions, with attendants and self-managers being the only people who "truly" understand the Direct Funding Program.

The real experts are the people with disabilities and their family members. Indeed, despite this study having a thread of anti-professional sentiment, it does not call for a *rejection* of expertise, but a *redefinition* of expertise. Adams (2010), in her historical review of professions in Canada, observes that as definitions evolve different occupations vie for inclusion, thus constantly stretching and reducing the parameters of what constitutes a profession. In the Direct Funding context, there is a push away from formal credentialed training, as people with disabilities are regarded as the experts in their needs, whereas attendants become experts in individual people. Arguably, an aspect of using the "attendant" terminology attributes status to this role. The attendants cultivate expertise in responding to the needs of specific individuals, and this expertise is gained on the job directly from a self-manager. Further, the broader necessity of professionals is not wholly denied, but linking "care" and "professional" attempts to limit the encroachment of professionals on the daily experiences of disability by more clearly identifying professional roles. Ironically, such a model echoes many feminist approaches to care, including the rationality of care (Waerness 1996), the logic of care (Mol 2006), and other ethics of care scholarship; however, this model may also undermine efforts to improve working conditions and attribute status to marginalized care workers.

Many of the participants admit there are certain skills in which self-managers cannot direct attendants. Self-manager Michael gives an example of when directing breaks down:

> I find there are a few things that I *can't* direct them, like we had a couple of people here who can't tie shoes, and I can't tell [them how] to tie a shoe because I've never tied one myself!

Jim explains how there are a few techniques and skills that might be taught formally in a classroom setting, but that the most important and challenging elements of being an attendant are more abstract:

> *Jim:* There are some good things [about PSW training], like they tell them how to [help us] live properly. There are a number of good things, how to clean properly, proper hygiene techniques.
> *CK:* But the philosophy isn't there?

Jim: The philosophy is that you're caring for a patient. What I'm trying to say is, you don't need it to be a good attendant. The experts will teach you. We have our own experts.

Being an Independent Living attendant is primarily a philosophical approach to disability that cannot be easily taught in a classroom setting and which has few transferable skills. Yet, many attendants in this study transition into work in related fields, such as physiotherapy or occupational therapy, or into more formalized attendant-service settings, eventually becoming a "care professional." From the outside (e.g., universities that have received their applications for a physiotherapy program), attendants may be read as paraprofessional care workers with experience, whereas within the Direct Funding Program, good attendants demonstrate an alternative positioning on disability and become important allies to people with disabilities. Many self-managers expressed disdain towards professionals, and particularly towards care and medical professionals, but they did not take issue with their attendants, friends, and family members working in these positions. Just like with Shauna's RN friend, it appears as though training in Independent Living philosophy is the primary transferable skill attendants gain, and such a perspective may be powerful enough to slowly change the meanings of care and medical professions from the inside out.

Illness, Medical Interventions, and Personal Care

The strong anti-professional and anti-medical messaging of Independent Living does not lead to advocating for the eradication of medical institutions but, as evidenced by attendants going on to become care professionals, to an implicit desire to change some of the foundational assumptions of these fields. Thus, although care is "not what happens here," it does not completely disappear. Two areas where care continues to apply are during times of illness and in reference to the most intimate aspects of attendant services.

The notion "We're not sick, we're disabled!" echoes throughout the history of disability movements in North America and resonates in contemporary Independent Living organizations and programming. It is important that people with disabilities are not assigned to the sick role in society, thereby excusing them from citizenship duties such as employment and decision making, decreasing expectations of and opportunities for their social participation, and culturally locating them on the fringes of society (DeJong 1983). The anti-medicalization thread in the disability movement is an important and powerful one, though it marginalizes the experiences of people who are sick with terminal, chronic, or acute curable diseases (e.g., people with HIV/AIDS or cancer) who might otherwise feel an affiliation with disability communities (Driedger and Owen 2008). In spite of the cultural and rhetorical significance of this message, many people with disabilities are prone to illnesses and sometimes have complex health issues.

In this study, there is a sense among participants that assistance during periods of illness and medical procedures can be considered care, and that these practices are never enjoyable but are necessary and must be tolerated. As Carolyn, an attendant, describes: "When it comes to care, I go to the hospital because ... I might need to be cared for in some kind of medical situation that I don't know about or that I'm unfamiliar with or that I don't have an expertise with." Care is a form of medical support where the person in need is often not feeling well and another person works to alleviate discomfort and assist the sick person to opt out of social responsibilities. This may require the expertise of a medical professional or, more commonly, assistance by a family member or friend. With the Independent Living approach, on the other hand, attendants help people with disabilities participate in life. This is a philosophical commitment: this study found that there are not enough attendant-service hours under the Direct Funding Program for self-managers to participate in all desired activities.

Self-managers and informal supports in particular recount crises of health, including bouts of serious injury, infection, surgeries, and complications from the underlying impairments of the self-managers. Detailed accounts of illness and injury emerged in thirty-six of the interviews. The detail and frequency of these narratives suggest their significance in the lives of the participants, as the interviews focused on attendant services and not on medical care. The Canadian Council on Social Development (2004, 1) finds that "persons with disabilities tend to have higher rates for a wide range of health conditions than do those without disabilities." Alongside their increased susceptibility to health conditions and narratives of health crises, participants insist on a distinction between medical needs and attendant care (i.e., "We're not sick, we're disabled"). For example, Jason, a self-manager, declares: "I don't have crazy medical requirements really. Um, not like on crazy machines, stuff like that. It's pretty straightforward stuff." Another self-manager, Ryan, similarly says: "I don't really have any underlying health problems or disability."

At first glance, it appears as though the distinction between crises of health (which require varied levels of informal and professional care) and the tasks of daily living (which require attendant services) can be clearly defined. This is reflected in the Ontario policy landscape, where attendant services are largely separated from primary care and medical home care. Victoria, a community advocate, talks about the difference between attendants and hospital workers:

[The committee I was involved in] was to assess whether the attendants' work was comparable to working in a hospital environment, and it's not, because of several factors. One is that *I'm* directing the work being done; my needs are routine, stable, life-long, self-directed, and they cease to be medical needs at that point. I don't need someone's trained judgment. I know what I need. Unless I get sick or I can't tell what I need – then I need nursing services, which are different from attendant services.

Thomas, a researcher with extensive community involvement, agrees and endorses the political separation of these functions, and helps articulate some of the ambivalence towards professionals:

A woman I know who has got a fabulous son – he's twelve years old – she needs a nurse three times a week for him because [his lungs get] clogged. He's got some very serious medical issues. He needs a nurse three times a week. But that's nursing care, or that's physiotherapy care, or whatever you want to call it. That care, it seems to me, should be a separate function but related to the life of the person, but not part of the individualized funding, so it should be separate funding. Because it's true, if a physiotherapist comes in ... because this is a specialized service, all I can do is tell the physiotherapist that I feel clogged in my chest. This person has studied for two years or four years or whatever. They're going to know what my chest needs, and they're going to recommend things to me. I can say yes or no. "Can I pat on your back?" "No, I don't want a pat on my back." So the person still has a say, but it's a little bit different, right?

Attendants assist with daily needs; professionals and informal supports help during temporary illness, depending on severity; and health professionals provide specialized services that may be needed on an occasional or regular basis.

The line between health needs requiring a care professional and everyday needs that can be managed by a self-manager and an attendant is not so clear from the point of view of the attendants, who are sometimes required to do tasks they do not feel qualified for. Long-term attendant Andrea notes:

Andrea: Even, sometimes it's really, almost medical, like the things that you
   have to do. You're surprised, [you think] that you're not qualified to do
   them. But it's still very informal.
CK: You think, "I can't believe I'm allowed to do this," is that what you mean?
Andrea: "I can't believe I've been asked to do this" sometimes.

For some self-managers, and implied by the current policy framework in Ontario, the distinction between attendant services and health needs is easy to identify, but it is the attendants who must navigate this fine line on a daily basis, sometimes resulting in their performing tasks that make them feel uncomfortable.

One aspect of the daily-needs component is categorized by interview participants as personal care. For example, self-manager Cheryl explains:

Cheryl: When I think of care, I think they, they have to turn me in bed, and
   when I go to bathroom, they have to wipe my butt. I hate that. But it
   has to be done. And I think that's care. Is that what you mean?
CK: Yeah. So you're not ...
Cheryl: It's personal.

Cheryl cuts me off and ends the conversation there. Personal care is necessary and is extremely private. These are the activities most commonly thought of in reference to care, that is, hands-on daily physical assistance with toileting, bathing, dressing, and grooming, and can be likened to Twigg's notion of body work (2000) or Tronto's "care-giving" phase of her definition of care (1993, 107). Personal care in this study is distinguished from help around the house, and even from help with eating. Personal care includes the daily routines that require touch and nudity, and the moments when self-managers feel the most vulnerable. Again, personal care is also the space where concerns about gender and sexual abuse arise for female self-managers. These activities are described in terms that go beyond intimate and are seen as the crux of attendant services.

During the most personal and perhaps complicated interactions, attendants must behave more formally than they do otherwise. The joking and the banter stop, as attendant Adam explains:

I guess at a certain point when you're doing something, let's say you're helping someone in the washroom, you might be talking with them beforehand

and it comes time to do some work, and I guess during that space of time both the client and the attendant sort of go into a space where this is a job that has to be done, and it's not pleasant and nobody likes it. The attendant doesn't like it and the client certainly doesn't like it, but it has to be done and it gets done. Then you go back to talking again. So maybe there is a space in there where that role becomes a little more black and white.

During these intimate moments, the attendant behaves professionally, perhaps temporarily becoming a semi-care professional. The most personal and concrete assistance is named and tolerated as a form of care.

The lines between illness, specialized interventions, and daily needs are sometimes ambiguous, yet a common place emerges where the formality and knowledge associated with professionals regain prominence and power. Certain activities, such as personal care or specialized health interventions, are too delicate, precarious, and intimate for the relaxed interacting sometimes associated with attendant work. The attendant or health professional is expected to focus, and the person in need reluctantly and temporarily enters the role of the patient in order to undergo physical interactions that can be uncomfortable and can be called "care." The informal working spaces of Direct Funding are not always relaxing; indeed, they can be distressing for the self-manager during personal care (recall Cheryl's "I hate that" in reference to being helped with her toileting needs) and help with medical needs. Self-managers and experienced attendants describe being formal with each other at the beginning of a relationship, and relaxing as they become more involved. If the required need is not physically painful or intimate – for example, help with cooking and eating – the attendants and self-managers are more likely to have informal, friendly interactions distanced from the idea of care.

Attendants can temporarily transform into semi-care professionals when providing personal care; in parallel, but more distressing for those involved, attendant services can transform into health care when the attendant-service system fails. Jennifer, a community advocate and self-manager, explains:

It was starting to look like I would end up going into a hospital because the service was falling apart, and you can't have it fall apart for very long. Like, how many days can you go without going to the washroom? Or without getting out of your chair and going to bed?

Isabelle, a self-manager, shares her crisis:

It's really, really tricky. So when I first [lived in a supported living arrangement, it] was not very good. The way they ran it wasn't very good. I don't
think they have it there anymore, actually. I just couldn't get the hours that
I needed ... so I ended up doing more physically than I should have been
doing and I got very sick ... I had a major flare-up.

These are not isolated experiences, as Independent Living employee Marie
makes clear when referring to Ontario's waiting list:

No, we don't jump [people in the waiting list] ... Well, I mean we jump once
in a while if there's a real crisis that we have to deal with right away. But
time is becoming more and more problematic because the longer people
wait, the closer they get to a crisis. So, I'd say the majority of the people on
the list are pretty much close to being in crisis.

Major failures of the system resulting in personal and physical crises are a
standard feature of the attendant-service landscape of Ontario, and a major
policy limitation of the current options for people with disabilities.

The concept of care continues to apply and is tolerated in reference to times
of illness and medical interventions, as well as to highly intimate personal care.
Care is permitted in these activities, and formality and professionalism are
drawn upon as tools to help ease the social discomfort around intimacy, autonomy, and bodies that misbehave. Care is also required when the attendant-service
system fails and self-managers experience personal and often physical crises of
health, collapsing the separation between health and attendant services.

Care and People with Intellectual Disabilities

The third bridge built by accessible care helps explore tensions and hierarchies
within disability studies and communities, namely tensions between people
with intellectual disabilities and people with physical disabilities. In the interview
process of this study, one of the earliest and most consistent themes that arose
is that care is for people with intellectual disabilities and for those who cannot
self-direct. This theme is particularly strong in the program information, which
stresses the need to self-direct and self-manage the attendant services, thereby
restricting those who cannot to more caring services options. Some participants'
comments reflect the tension between self-advocates with physical disabilities
and people with intellectual disabilities and their supports (Douglas 2010b;
Ryan and Runswick-Cole 2008; Hillyer 1993). Several self-managers proudly

commented on "only" having a physical impairment, while informal supports spoke of the relief they felt upon learning that the self-managers had no apparent intellectual impairment as young children. For example, one commented her child's eyes being "bright, intelligent; there was no dullness." Other remarks were more directly offensive to people with intellectual disabilities. For example, in reference to whether the Direct Funding Program could work for people who may not be able to self-direct as it is currently defined, one self-manager said: "Well, I guess if they have intellectual disability, I mean, you have watch them [so] they don't set fire to the couch kind of thing." Many of the attendants expressed discomfort, either in theory or based on practice, about working with people with intellectual disabilities, as they were concerned about knowing what to do if the person could not direct verbally.

The picture being presented is troubling. In the context of this program, care is not acceptable for those receiving or working under Direct Funding, but it is acceptable for "them," that is, people who cannot self-direct. Reg, an ally and community-based researcher, muses:

> I still think that people with intellectual disabilities are at risk of being looked down upon because rationality is so highly prized in our society. You know, "I've got my mind, dear," you know? It's like so foundational to how we conceive of the human person that any kind of detraction of that is sometimes perceived as a diminishment of a person's humanity, which I don't believe, but that's the way things often get played out. So, there's probably vestiges of that that are still there ... within the disability community, as in the society more generally.

This study revealed a derision of people with intellectual disabilities and a valorization of rationality and independence. As mentioned, the participants representing the intellectual disability community also distanced themselves from the idea of care, which suggests that the critiques of care are not limited to people with physical disabilities and reveals schisms in Ontario disability spheres. It is unfortunate to report on this ongoing tension and evidence of discrimination in the heart of a movement that seeks inclusion and social rights for people with disabilities, especially when there are similar programs accommodating people with intellectual disabilities (most notably in the United Kingdom). People with intellectual disabilities are not allowed in Ontario's Independent Living–run Direct Funding Program, raising important questions for the future and present status of disability movements in the province.

Significantly, many of the participants' responses when asked if Direct Funding should be expanded to include people with intellectual disabilities highlighted gaps in the current administration that would make it untenable, and the strain of the program's long waiting list. For example, disability leader Jim says:

> [Supporting people with intellectual disabilities is] a totally different concept. You have to care for somebody who can't care for themselves. The thing about care, I know you're interested in that, is it only comes up in the one situation where you mentioned, [that is for] the parents of children or adults with intellectual disabilities. That was the one place where it came up, and they were after us quite a few times to allow their people onto our model, but it doesn't fit.

The program is designed in such a way that excludes people with intellectual disabilities from accessing it. Since the program is so closely linked to advocacy and Independent Living, this exclusion reinforces divisions within disability communities and movements. Nick, a self-manager, sums up the main tension:

> *CK:* Do you think it changes if, if [people with intellectual disabilities] are allowed in?
> *Nick:* Yeah! I thought you had to self-manage!
> *CK:* Well, you do right now; they haven't changed it.
> *Nick:* I think they, they should call it something else.

The program is not just a policy mechanism that delivers funds but is a manifestation of Independent Living philosophy. The program is not about receiving funds but about individual autonomy and is contingent upon a narrow understanding of Independent Living.

Despite this clear distinction, the consensus is that people with intellectual disabilities *should* have access to a similar sort of program, with the right safeguards and mechanisms in place (and there are similar programs through the Ontario Ministry of Community and Social Services). For example, Joel, an Independent Living employee, notes:

> I think Direct Funding as a model can work. I think for people with disabilities, it should be them in control first and foremost. If they can't be in control, there could be supports set up ... whether that's the parents,

whether that's Adult Protective Service Workers, whether an informal support circle could be developed and a structure supported so that that happens.

Developing infrastructure and safeguards is an important detail because it unsettles the logic linking oppression and people with intellectual disabilities. By containing care to certain areas, the participants change its meanings in an attempt to diminish the oppressive potentials of care. Providing care for people who cannot make decisions independently or completely self-direct as defined by Independent Living does not grant permission for abuse or even encroachment on their agency. The participants acknowledge that, from certain angles, the current program is exclusionary, inadequate, and perhaps oppressive in its own way. The multiple and contested meanings of care are starkly apparent, as it can mean an oppressive attitude towards people with physical disabilities in one instance, and a form of exclusion of people with intellectual disabilities in another. Removing care from Direct Funding and containing it requires us to develop appropriate forms of (not) care for the people it excludes, perhaps encouraging critical reflection on the limits of Independent Living.

Implications of Removing Care

As explored in Chapter 1, recent scholarship engaging feminist and disability perspectives seeks to explain the tensions and identify mutual "passionate commitments" (Watson et al. 2004, 341). This literature documents a polemic between the independent, masculinist approach of disability movements, which completely eliminates and devalues care, and the feminist, interdependent approaches, often focusing on the ethics of care. For example, Hughes and colleagues (2005, 263 and 264) note: "The [Disabled People's Movement] has adopted a pragmatic and materialist interpretation of care that is commensurate with its masculinist ethics and idealizes masculinist notions of autonomy," and

> feminist theorists, by contrast, argue that the dominant model of the "worker citizen" obscures the need for, and the potential of, the "carer citizen." The carer citizen also works but she will be drawn into emotional and pragmatic relations of interdependency, invariably and in embodied ways, throughout the life-course, most likely as both a carer and a worker.

This work goes on to argue that the approaches are not as disparate as they seem and that the confrontational tone in some articles (e.g., Silvers 1997) and actual confrontations at academic conferences (Thomas 2007) may be overstated, as there are places of common ground, including connections to social movements, shared concern with "the problem of caring work" (Watson et al. 2004, 341), revised definitions of independence, and inclusion of the concepts of citizenship, justice, and rights (Kröger 2009, 415–16). Yet, most authors seem to conclude that the feminist approaches to care are more holistic than Independent Living, which is depicted as limited. For example, Watson and colleagues (2004, 340) declare, "The solution lies, we argue, in exploring the emancipatory potential of the concept of interdependence." In this study, however, the process of controlling what care means is an effort to reduce its oppressive potentials, incorporate specific histories, and move inter/dependence to appropriate spheres in life. This effort does not fully succeed, as demonstrated by tensions with intellectual disability communities, but it does begin to alter the terms of the theoretical debates between feminist and disability scholars.

Many feminist care researchers argue that focusing on independence, as happens in Independent Living, masks the interdependency of our social worlds, or "inevitable dependencies" as Kittay (1999, 14) claims (see also Arneil 2009). Containing care to particular worlds does not mask inter/dependence but moves it. Moving care refers to containing the meanings of care in order to highlight the oppressive potential and specific histories of disability linked to the concept, yet without denying that care must still take place at times, and has transformative potential. As such, moving care as represented by the Direct Funding Program is one way care can be "made accessible." This move sometimes results in the removal of the notions of care and interdependency from public documents linked to Independent Living, but it does not deny the value of these concepts. The spaces of inevitable dependencies, where care is required, are reserved and respected. There is potential to use these spaces to engage deeply with other oppressive histories linked to care. Self-managers reluctantly enter these spaces when necessary – in times of health crisis, for specialized medical treatments, or daily during the most intimate personal care, sometimes accompanied by an attendant and at other times by a health professional. Independence and interdependency, care/not care, are not in competition but flash in and out of prominence depending on the circumstance, relationship, life stage, and individual. Although the theoretical literature documents a debate *between* independence and interdependence, in which interdependence often seems to win out, this oversimplifies the cultural, political, and material effects of the Independent Living message.

For feminist care scholars, part of revaluing care as a gendered form of labour is recognizing the oppressive sides of it. Nirmala Erevelles (2011, 190) persuasively argues, "In highlighting the exploitative nature of caring work ... [feminist political economists'] analyses have placed disabled persons, who are of course central to this debate, as antagonistic to the interests of the class, race, and gender politics." For Erevelles, feminist political economists overwhelmingly overlook the historical and material conditions that create "the 'other' side of the dialectic," that is, notions of disability, dependency, and social welfare, even while carefully attending to the histories and politics of race, class, and so on. Willingness to incorporate critiques of care and histories relevant to disability echoes feminist reflexivity and does not denigrate care, but rather represents it as the complex tension it is. Disability perspectives seek to challenge and reveal what Tronto (1993, 6) terms "moral boundaries" – "ideas [that] function as boundaries to exclude some ideas of morality from consideration." Tronto does not seek to dismantle all boundaries, but rather to redraw them. Disability perspectives participate in redrawing the boundaries around care in order to facilitate the urgent recognition of the less favourable aspects. Feminist care scholarship, in its own way, can express a form of what Tronto (1993, 120–21) terms "privileged irresponsibility" or "the opportunity simply to ignore certain forms of hardships that they do not face." That is, refusing to acknowledge the histories of oppression and ongoing abuses that are *also* linked to care alongside racialized, gendered, and classed histories. Of course, disability perspectives must also consider the implications for worker rights, access to services by people with intellectual disabilities, and so on. Moving care contains its meanings and facilitates this critical and essential process.

Closing Thoughts

In the exploration of what care is not and what care is, the meaning of care that resonates the strongest is as an outlook on disability with the potential to lead to experiences of oppression. In this context, care is not merely the concrete body work, nor is it the relational negotiation that takes place between attendants and people with disabilities, even if we sometimes use the term "care" to describe these items. This is a clear political message that condemns speaking for others, the power of the medical institution, and pity for and the regulating of disabled people to the margins of society. Rhetorically pushing care into certain realms shifts the focus to the broader social and cultural exclusions linked to care, asserting, 'This is not what we do here.' Care, in the agency-denying, abusive, oppressive sense, is no longer an all-encompassing response to disability but is limited, and its power differentials are levelled in some aspects. Limiting the meanings of care does not undermine the universal experience of dependency, as highlighted by feminist scholars such as Kittay (1999). Instead, as feminist ethicists note, it reminds us to attend to the particular, situated, embodied experiences of giving and receiving support. Certainly, saying that "care" applies to people with intellectual disabilities does not mean that abuse or institutionalization is condoned, but rather acknowledges that there are instances where someone, perhaps a care professional or family member, must speak on behalf of someone who cannot always do so, at least not in conventional ways. Moving care does not provide all the answers; this is clear particularly in light of exclusions of people with intellectual disabilities from certain aspects of Independent Living movements.

Independence, as manifested through consumer direction and a rejection of care, does not universally "win" under the Direct Funding Program; instead, it is reasserted as an important value that disabled people should have access to. Direct Funding creates the conditions for independence to be expressed in relationship with others, most often attendants. Meanwhile, the spaces where care still takes place are also changed; the oppressive potentials diminish (though are not eliminated) by containing care and reducing the authority and reach of the medical institution and professionals. Theoretical literature on care must thus account for the disability critiques and attempt to discern what the removal of care means both for attendant services and for the arenas where care is transformed or deemed appropriate and left intact.

PART 3

Policy and Social Movement Implications

5

Intricate Messages, Local and Transnational Erasures

Disability scholarship and Ontario's Direct Funding Program attempt to *do* something by distancing from the concept of care. Distinguishing attendant services from other forms of home care, and attempting to contain and redefine its more theoretical meanings, are not accidental or arbitrary. Removing care from the program materials is an intentional strategy to improve the daily experiences of disability that are in the shadow of more institutionalized approaches to care. The messages about care in the Direct Funding Program serve as signposts for promoting changes to the daily, lived experiences of people with physical disabilities enrolled in this program. But this unique strategy also has unintended consequences in policy realms outside the program.

The rhetorical removal of care has implications not just for seemingly abstract theoretical discussions about care among academic feminist and disability scholars but for numerous ongoing policy discussions. Challenging our understandings of care can obscure other policy issues, namely the limitations of the program, the availability of disability supports, and transnational issues. Yet, it also conveys a nuanced message that can potentially change current policy conversations in transformative ways, thus showing the far-reaching effects of the removal of care.

The rhetorical removal of care from the Direct Funding Program obfuscates other policy issues. First, the mandatory relational work of direct funding instills an unusually strong sense of obligation in the attendants that in some ways hides limitations of the program. The relational ontologies help frame the work environment as "not like work" and create an informality that is highly valued by attendants while changing their expectations of working conditions. Second, the availability of services can be obscured by the "arms and legs" characterization of attendants, which resonates with the rationale behind accessibility legislation, such as the Accessibility for Ontarians with Disabilities Act (Bill 118 2005). Finally, the removal of care contributes to the transnational erasure of individuals who cross borders and end up working as attendants, or using the services themselves.

"Moving" care to certain areas creates complex messages that overwhelm the policy landscape. Reserving care for professionals while rejecting the power they hold leads to an ambiguous and nuanced position regarding professionalism. This has implications for the push to professionalize attendants through standardized personal support worker training and discussions on provincial regulation of these workers (Laporte and Rudoler 2013; Kelly and Bourgeault 2015). Further, seeing care as tied to health and intimate needs reveals the limitations of a social/health policy divide, with implications for which Ontario ministry houses the Direct Funding Program. Although these messages do not fully register in present discussions, they serve as placeholders that can potentially change policy discussions in interesting ways.

Obscuring Program Limitations and Availability of Services

Several known and new limitations of the Direct Funding Program emerged in this study, including attendant salaries being different depending on the setting, and the difficulties in recruiting and retaining attendants, especially for short or overnight shifts. Participants suggested increasing or even doubling the hourly wage and compensating attendants for mileage as the most immediate ways of improving the program. Self-managers complained about the amount of administrative work required, the length of the waiting list (four to five years at the time of the study), and the application process being dated (e.g., instructions to use a typewriter). Two of the most urgent limitations of the Direct Funding Program have links to the mandatory relational work (framed as "not care") that attendants and self-managers participate in, namely the cap on hours and the need for reliable back-up support. Self-managers foster *caring* relationships to encourage attendants to provide emergency back-up support or to work extra hours when needed; attendants are also fuelled by genuine attachment to the self-managers and concern for their well-being. Categorizing this aspect of Direct Funding as "not care" and as optional obscures the shortfalls of the program.

When the data was collected for this study, the Direct Funding Program allowed for a daily maximum of six hours of attendant services, although this has since been raised to seven. Exceptions, including extra hours for people using ventilators, access to an emergency fund during times of acute illness, and extra hours to support self-managers with young children, are made on a case-by-case basis (CILT 2000). The daily maximum does not affect allocation of additional home care hours for specialized medical needs, such as treatment of pressure sores, which can be arranged separately through local Community Care Access Centres. In many cases, up to six hours a day is sufficient, especially for self-managers who live with another self-manager (such as a spouse or room-mate), where it's possible to pool hours for shared services during mealtimes. Some self-managers in this situation would like to be able to combine their funding in a joint bank account or go through the Direct Funding Program interview together, which might be an interesting proposal for CILT to consider. However, for other self-managers who live on their own, the six-hour limit can be quite restrictive. The first areas to cut back on are recreational activities, social events, and travel; ironically, improved access to these types of activities is cited as one of the key benefits of this style of service delivery (Parker et al. 2000; Roeher Institute 1997). One self-manager explains, "[I need to] fill in the gaps of Direct Funding because I don't have enough funding to go work out or go play [sports]." Self-managers must, in key informant Marie's words, "pick and choose" what they use their hours for. Another self-manager explains:

With six [hours], think [I'm] about two short a day give or take. Certain days are worse than others. Fridays are good days for me, I play wheelchair [sports] on Friday nights. That's two hours alone. Saturdays would be nice as well. It would be nice to be able to go grocery shopping, something I'm not able to do [with my current number of hours].

The Direct Funding Program had limited increases in capital between 1998 and 2011, when the pilot program became a full-fledged program (Parker et al. 2000). When the Ontario government announced an expansion of the program in 2014, it included a slight increase in maximum hours, but the eligibility criteria remained the same (CILT 2014). Marie and others in this study note that the needs of people with disabilities can increase over time because of aging or progressive impairments, requiring self-managers to do more with the same number of attendant-service hours. The program administrators must be vigilant about the fixed amount of money: giving one self-manager more hours means that potential users will remain on the waiting list longer, thereby increasing the potential for a crisis. Unfortunately for both the administrators and the users of the program, it is a zero-sum system.

Community advocate and self-manager Jennifer makes an important clarification about attendant-service hours:

> There's a concern that every person with a disability is automatically going to want twenty-four hours of people around. So there's this fear that it will be an endless request, like a bottomless pit of requests, but I don't think so, because you also want your privacy and you also want your own time. You don't want to have an attendant with you constantly ... Most people will just ask for what they need, and that's all they'll ask for.

In this study, self-managers greatly appreciate attendants and see them as important people in their lives, but they also want to maintain a semblance of privacy, particularly the self-managers with families (see also Malacrida 2009).

Some self-managers fill in the gaps through work-based accommodations, whereas others informally rely on co-workers, friends, family, and even strangers; continuing to rely on informal supports while using Direct Funding was also documented in the early evaluation of the pilot project (Roeher Institute 1997). Many self-managers insisted they did not want their informal supports included as participants in this study, perhaps downplaying the inadequacies of the program. Most commonly, self-managers in the study draw on the relational component of attendant services to fill in the gaps. Self-managers work hard to build rapport and instill a deep sense of obligation in their attendants, sometimes resulting in attendants working without pay. For example, as attendant Madison says:

> If you're doing the bedtime shift, then it makes up for [working extra earlier in the day]; if you're not, then it does kinda feel like I just did an extra half hour of work that I'm not getting paid for. If I was working [at] McDonald's, I wouldn't even do that, I'd just walk out. But you know, it's different because [the self-manager is] a buddy.

Long-term attendant Rob explains how the relationships are his primary reason for working under Direct Funding, a job that is not "an ideal system":

> I helped two friends of mine who had disabilities who received Direct Funding largely because they needed the assistance. I didn't mind going to

visit my friends, so to speak, and I just went and also helped them out because they needed the assistance. But quite frankly, I don't think it's an ideal system, only because it's hard to find staff to work such short shifts.

The same sense of obligation based on relationship is drawn upon to avoid instances where self-managers are stranded and reminded of their vulnerabilities. Attendant Melissa recounts:

> *Melissa:* There was one day that [the self-manager] calls me, it's like at one
> o'clock in the morning. He's like, "My attendant hasn't showed up yet,
> can you come put me to bed?" ... So I get out of bed, I get dressed, I
> start going. I'm on the [bus and he] calls me again, "Oh, don't bother
> coming. My attendant just showed up." I was like –
> *CK:* Thanks.
> *Melissa:* Fuck! So I jumped off the bus, went back home, and back to bed.
> It's things like that, you can't just leave them stranded, right?

Melissa goes above and beyond what she would do in other work settings, to ensure that the self-manager is properly supported. Self-manager Ryan articulates the connection between relationships and the gaps of the program:

> I'm not going to like everything everybody does, because everyone has their
> own little way of doing it. And if I start nagging at them to do it my way,
> then we lose that friendship. And it would become more of an employee-
> employer relationship. They will only come in for that hour and a half, and
> leave right away. Whereas if we develop a rapport or a friendship, if I want
> to eat a little more dinner ... then we can do that and I won't feel bad about
> keeping them a little more.

Feminist researchers have long discussed the distinctions and connections between "caring for" and "caring about" (Grant et al. 2004). In this study, cultivated caring or emotional attachments can be drawn upon to compensate for a shortage in hours or to prevent experiences of vulnerability. Excluding the concept of care from public rhetoric of the Direct Funding Program obscures this strategy to some extent. Caring relationships are transformed into an integral component of the daily operations of the program and make it appear to be running more efficiently than it actually is; this component is difficult to account for or to commodify in discussions of care work (Lynch, Baker, and Lyons 2009), especially when care is so fervently rejected in the public discourse.

Relational Ontology and the Evaluation of Working Conditions

The relational ontologies created under Direct Funding, categorized as "not care," can be linked to the attendants' lack of critical evaluation of their working conditions. Many attendants, particularly young attendants who work or have worked for self-managers of a similar age, expressed that their jobs are "not like work." For example, attendant Kristina says, "[I'd go] grocery shopping and do some cooking, and I'd vacuum or something, but, we talked a lot and we got along really well, so it didn't feel like work and I didn't dread going." Attendant Adam concurs: "Sometimes it doesn't seem like a job at all ... After a while, you're going to hang out with your friends and every once in a while they need a hand." Similarly, attendant Hailey says: "It actually worked out really well because we ended up being friends; it didn't really even feel like a job." This was a strong theme, particularly among attendants who worked while doing post-secondary education, and is a part of why the attendants enjoy this type of work. Self-manager Jason explains how the sense of "not like work" may be intentionally cultivated:

> I like the informality of it. It does not [have to be] really strict, like the casual nature of it. Because that's my house, you know? I don't want my house to feel like a place of work, even though it is.

Self-managers want to maintain a sense of home to help temper the feeling of being "on" all the time when attendants are present. Self-managers work diligently to create a relaxed, informal work environment, one in which the attendants also feel at ease. The home environment contributes to the informality of attendant work, which is further established through the relational ontology of attendant work, in the spaces between the attendants and the self-managers. The relational ontologies of attendant work starkly contrast the independent worker model employed in many contemporary work settings, and help prevent attendant services from medicalization. Many of the attendants in this study and in others value the relationships they form with self-managers; however, a caregiver in England's (2010, 144) study of Canada's Live-in Caregiver Program "clearly despises the 'part of the family' rhetoric which [the participant] interpreted as a strategy of extracting further unpaid physical and affective labour, without the genuine caring and respect associated with actual familial relationships." Indeed, cultivating and drawing on relationships within home settings to fill in the gaps of inadequate social programs is a practice potentially exploitative of workers.

The sense of "not like work" extends beyond the attendants' personal reflections and the self-managers' efforts. In a discussion of the wage gap between Direct Funding attendants and attendants employed in other settings, Aaron, from the Ontario Ministry of Health and Long-Term Care, explains:

> Even though a self-manager is employing attendants, it's not considered to be a "workplace" for the purposes of the pay equity legislation. So, in the same way that the workers working for an individual can't organize a union, for example, it's considered [that] the classification of a worker under the Direct Funding Program is really basically the same as a domestic [worker] – you know, if you're hiring a nanny, if you're hiring somebody to work in your own home. So, it's a class of workers that were excluded from pay equity legislation.

The resulting informal work environment protects the sense of home for the self-manager and is an appealing feature of the work for attendants; however, it unintentionally maintains the status quo of the material working conditions. Lilly (2008) argues that the home environment contributes to the feminization and financial devaluation of home care work in contrast to more medical settings. England (2010, 314) observes, "Because the home is viewed primarily as a site of 'non-work,' any waged work occurring there is liable to be viewed as secondary or supplemental." The sense of "not like work," in combination with isolation from other attendants, means the expectations for other work environments do not seem to apply.

Although many self-managers stressed the need to increase wages in order to attract and keep attendants, many of the attendants expressed satisfaction with the wages. For example, attendant Jillian notes:

> I thought [the pay] was great [laugh]! I don't remember exactly what it was. I want to say it was around $13 an hour or somewhere in that vicinity. But it was definitely more than minimum wage, which is what I would be getting probably anywhere else I had worked at the time. So, yeah, I thought it was fantastic.

The attendants' satisfaction is possibly connected to how they see this work within their career plans. Attendant work is seen as temporary, something "on the side." The majority of study participants were students when they worked as attendants and had access to medical and dental benefits through their postsecondary institutions, parents, or partners. Attendant work thus becomes the "perfect job for a student," as Jillian says. Indeed, twelve of the fifteen attendants interviewed started (and some finished) working as attendants while attending postsecondary institutions. Eight self-managers cited advertising at colleges and universities as a recruitment strategy. The variable hours were seen as an advantage to attendants, as they could fit them among school obligations. Madison sums up this situation: "I think it's pretty fair, and I don't have any complaints. But, on the other hand, I don't live off it." The 1997 pilot project evaluation notes that 74 percent of attendants surveyed had begun postsecondary education, with 47 percent completing a college diploma or university degree (Roeher Institute 1997, 51). Although dated, these numbers may suggest that the sample in this study is skewed; however, the numbers may also suggest that the demographic has changed since the pilot and that the workers Direct Funding attracts are different from those in other care settings. For example, in a preliminary survey of Ontario personal support workers (PSWs), Lum, Sladek, and Ying (2010) found that 96 percent are women, and 76 percent are forty years old or older, which is quite distinct from the attendants in this study (see also Lyon and Glucksmann 2008).

At one point, nine attendants in this study earned income solely from Direct Funding; this was unsustainable for them and they ended up moving on or piecing together additional work in both related and unrelated fields. Not one of the attendants could work under Direct Funding as a primary means of income for a sustained period. I am not convinced that the fear of attendants being drawn away from Direct Funding jobs into more institutionalized care settings (commonly cited in reports and advocacy comparing wages and benefits; for example, see OCSA 2008) is founded, again suggesting that attendants comprise a group different from what is reported for PSWs in Ontario. Lum, Sladek, and Ying (2010, 7) argue that there are indications that PSWs are "committed to their work as a career path as opposed to a short term job," documenting that 44 percent have worked in the field for ten years or more. Only three attendants in this study seemed to be making a career out of attendant work, but worked in other attendant settings in addition to their Direct Funding obligations. Most of the attendants specifically liked the informality and flexibility of working under Direct Funding (for a limited period, anyway) and did not necessarily intend to work in other long-term care arrangements.

The apparent satisfaction with relatively unsatisfactory material working conditions (the subjective, relational benefits and informal environment were seen as job perks) helps cement the anti-union sentiments towards the Direct Funding Program. Reports and information on Direct Funding seem to discourage unionization, perhaps overstating the impact this might have on the program. A historic tension exists between Ontario unions and Independent Living, including Direct Funding advocates (Cranford 2005). Some advocates identify limitations with unionized workers and downplay the possibility that self-managers might be abusive (e.g., Parker et al. 2000, 16). For example, in a report published in 2000, organized labour is identified as a barrier to the establishment of the program, with no anticipated resolution (Yoshida et al. 2000). According to the authors, "In prior years, there have been consumers who have complained about problems encountered with unionized workers, for example, refusing to lift or transfer them"; the report implies that the concerns of organized labour are unfounded, since self-managers are "vulnerable employers" (25 and 26). The concept of vulnerable employers suggests that disabled people are incapable of abuse and exploitation, which does not fit with the findings of this study. For example, one key informant explains:

[The unions are] really vicious, mean people who threatened to fight against the program because, when pushed to the wall for the reason why, they said, "Because we cannot trust you not to abuse these attendants." So, they're accusing us disabled, hapless, paralyzed people who are absolutely dependent for our life and going to the bathroom and everything else, of being potential abusers of the staff!

It was unexpected to hear the terms "hapless" and "absolutely dependent" while interviewing key informants in Independent Living. This rhetoric was a marked shift from the more commonly used discourses of empowerment and independence, a shift that arose only in discussions of unions. Attendants in multiple environments are vulnerable to abuse (Armstrong et al. 2011), though not nearly as vulnerable as are self-managers (Matthias and Benjamin 2003; Saxton et al. 2001). Another example:

If [unionization] did happen, I think, from the consumer end, I think we'd be back to that situation where we'd be in the fallout of labour disruptions and that kind of thing. We'd be held hostage for that kind of thing, because people are in their own homes, they'd be all the more vulnerable to being abandoned if somebody just walked out and couldn't help them – or if they were on strike, people would be extremely vulnerable because how would you get around to do the basics for people?

Yoshida and colleagues (2000, 26) claim that the concerns of labour were "positively addressed" by the 1997 program evaluation, though they don't make clear the specifics of the resolution.

Cobble and Merrill (2008, 154) argue that service workers "are the future of trade unionism." It is integral, they suggest, to use nontraditional organizing strategies that, in the case of the Direct Funding Program, may help dispel the stereotypes and resistance to unionization. Drawing on the example of home care workers who organized in California, Cobble and Merrill (2008, 162) highlight the importance of "creating a unionism which could help solve the problems of both service producers and service consumers," thereby supporting an approach that would ensure the provision of ongoing attendant services during labour disruptions. Unionization is only one possible option for improving working conditions as well as the quality of service for disabled people under the Direct Funding Program; however, the anti-union sentiments may stifle discussions about working conditions.

Graduate students in the field of disability studies, along with a coalition made up of and representing people with intellectual disabilities living in group homes, articulate a nuanced perspective (Rinaldi and Walsh 2011), one which arose from the unionized developmental service workers who undertook strike action outside the group homes where they worked. Rinaldi and Walsh (2011, n.p.) explain:

[Bill 23, the Protecting Vulnerable People against Picketing Act] honours union members' right to strike, yet would prohibit striking at a particular kind of location. An inappropriate location would be outside the homes of people with intellectual disabilities, those who during the '07 and '09 strikes reported feeling antagonized, unable to leave their homes, and incapable of daily living when replacement workers were delayed from getting to work on time, all due to picket lines on the premises.

As is further discussed later, at times the Direct Funding Program can diverge from intellectual disability developments in other policy spheres. The informality of attendant work is seen as an important job perk but also creates the sense of "not like work," shifting the focus away from attempts to change the material working conditions and potentially drawing more students into this work than into other attendant settings. Aside from obscuring some of the specific limitations of the Direct Funding Program, the rhetorical removal of care can also obscure broader availability of disability supports.

The AODA and "Arms and Legs"

As part of the removal of care, attendants are frequently characterized as self-managers' "arms and legs." In this discourse, attendants become disembodied replacement parts that can correct unaccommodating environments. An attendant corrects, as Garland-Thomson (2011, 594) terms it, a "misfit," and facilitates a "fit," which "occurs when a harmonious, proper interaction occurs between a particularly shaped and functioning body and an environment that sustains that body." As long as attendants are available and familiar with Independent Living philosophy, they can help mitigate the social and physical effects of disability. Positioning attendants as "arms and legs" helps emphasize the necessity of their work (i.e., as necessary as an arm) but objectifies attendants to some extent – a criticism often levelled against disability perspectives on care (Thomas 2007). Further, the functional emphasis draws attention away from the availability and adequacy of attendant services.

This unintended consequence can also be seen in the efforts of various Ontario and national groups from the disability sector that were centrally involved in establishing the Accessibility for Ontarians with Disabilities Act (AODA). This legislation sets out to "achieve accessibility for Ontarians with disabilities with respect to goods, services, facilities, accommodation, employment, buildings, structures and premises on or before January 1, 2025" through the development and implementation of standards in five arenas with which the private, nonprofit, and public sectors are legally obligated to comply (Bill 118 2005). This is markedly different from earlier approaches to disability policy in Canada (Chivers 2007; Neufeldt 2003) and resonates with the Americans with Disabilities Act, in the United States. The first standard, the Accessibility Standard for Customer Service, has been in effect for the public sector since 2010, with the remaining standards rolling out in an integrated format over the next ten years (Ontario Ministry of Community and Social Services 2011). The legislation does not, however, have a clear strategy for enforcement.

The AODA is an ambitious and urgent undertaking, and the topic of attendants (termed "support persons" in the document) occasionally comes up. Linked to characterizing attendants as "arms and legs," the AODA presumes that attendant services are already in place, and operating smoothly and effectively. For example, in the customer service standard, support persons are discussed in section 4, grouped together with service animals (Accessibility Standards for Customer Service 2007). Resonating with the "arms and legs" framework, attendants and service animals are framed as assistive technology that correct inaccessible environments and mitigate disability. Regarding transportation, the AODA's Integrated Accessibility Standards declares:

> No conventional transportation service provider and no specialized transportation service provider shall charge a fare to a support person who is accompanying a person with a disability where the person with a disability has a need for a support person. (Integrated Accessibility Standards Regulation 2011, section 38.1)

It is assumed that support people are available to travel for short or long distances with the person they are supporting, and presumably are paid to do so. In reality, the Direct Funding Program and other arrangements have long waiting lists, with the Attendant Services Advisory Committee reporting a four- to ten-year wait across all types of attendant service options (OCSA 2008). For those who do have access to attendant services, many of the options are tied to the building in which they are delivered (with the exception of Direct Funding). This study found that, even with Direct Funding, self-managers did not have enough attendant-service hours for many activities deemed extra, including accompaniment on local transportation and overnight trips (see also Church, Diamond, and Voronka 2004).

Charles Beer, in his independent review of the AODA (2010, 16), comments:

> Let me make an observation concerning the availability and importance of American Sign Language (ALS) interpreters and Langue des signes québécoise (LSQ) interpreters, real time captioners and attendant care workers. In my own consultations we experienced challenges in scheduling sessions as a result of the limited supply of these necessary services across the province. It became clear to me that it is critical for these resources to be available in order to make it possible for people with various disabilities to fully participate in public forums, especially where the issues being discussed relate directly to accessibility. As we move to 2025, strategies to increase the supply of these critical human resources need be considered.

Here, Beer identifies a glaring oversight in the AODA's sweeping, multisector approach. How can Ontario be considered accessible by 2025 if the necessary services are unavailable or have long waiting lists attached to them? Calls for more and improved services come from outside work regarding the AODA and the Direct Funding Program, as seen in efforts to establish a Canadians with Disabilities Act and work related to the UN Convention of the Rights of Persons with Disabilities.[1] Further, in Ontario, CILT and other community stakeholders established the Attendant Services Advisory Committee through the Ontario Community Support Association to advocate for issues related to attendant services (OCSA 2008). This work takes place *separately* from the Direct Funding Program and from the galvanization around the AODA. Indeed, by framing attendants as "arms and legs" who do not perform care, attendants become assistive devices, and discussing access to these devices is thus out of the purview for many disability-related organizations, policies, legislation, and government ministries.

Transnational Erasures

The fourth bridge in accessible care highlights connections between the local and the transnational, and how the emphasis on choice and control incorporated into the removal of care from the Direct Funding Program supersedes transnational issues. A preliminary survey of Ontario personal support workers documents a high proportion of racialized women working in long-term care settings: 42 percent of the surveyed workforce, in contrast to the 23 percent of the total provincial population they constitute (Lum, Sladek, and Ying 2010). Less well documented, many of these women are first-generation Canadians (Zeytinoglu and Muteshi 1999).[2] Many feminist scholars highlight a globalized trend of transnational care-worker migration that is at play in the Canadian context (Mahon and Robinson 2011; Parreñas 2008; Zimmerman, Litt, and Bose 2006). Arlie Hochschild (2000) terms this trend a "global care chain" where women from the Global South migrate to the Global North to fill the care deficit caused by two-income households and the aging population, and in order to send home remittances. Migrating care workers thus directly alter the economies of their home countries and also end up conscripting other women with even more limited socioeconomic opportunities to look after the children and family

---

[1] Calls for a national act have diminished, with the exception of a small Ontario group with an independent advocate, Scott Allardyce, at the helm (Scott Allardyce, pers. comm.). Most other Canadian disability groups, including the Council of Canadians with Disabilities, shifted focus to the UN Convention on the Rights of Persons with Disabilities, which has the potential to serve a similar function to a national act.

[2] A 2006 Statistics Canada survey found that immigrants fill approximately 22 percent of the positions in "health occupations" (Statistics Canada 2011). This number does not clearly indicate the number of immigrant *care workers*, as it does not distinguish between varied types of health professionals. As well, the survey makes a distinction between social and health occupations, which is a blurred line in attendant services and other forms of home care.

members left behind. Further, many people with disabilities are denied entry into Canada because of unflinchingly exclusionary immigration policies. These invisible bodies never enter policy discussions of waiting lists and availability of attendant services. There are also, of course, countless people worldwide who are living with disabilities and impairments that are a direct result of the actions of Canada and other countries in the Global North (Soldatic 2013). The economic and social dynamics of the globalized care chain are significant, and the ongoing tensions of colonialism, gender, and race play out in daily interactions and in the geopolitical arena (Glenn 2010). This reflects the broader critique by Meekosha (2011, 668) (and other authors) of much of disability studies scholarship; she argues: "Disability studies was constructed as a field of knowledge without reference to the theorists, or the social experiences, of the global south."

In this study, three attendants declined to participate because of their discomfort with the English language, and some of the self-managers spoke about their experiences hiring immigrants as attendants. There is no current comprehensive demographic data of Direct Funding attendants; however, the 1997 evaluation of the program documents only 16 percent of attendants as visible minorities and only 10 percent whose first language is neither English or French (with a likely overlap between these two figures) (Roeher Institute 1997). The misaligned numbers from the PSW survey again suggest that there may be a different demographic profile of attendants working under Direct Funding in comparison with other settings. Yet, this preliminary evidence does indicate that the Ontario attendant-service sector is also implicated in the global care chain to some degree. The identity dynamics that may result are alluded to in community documents on attendant services and Direct Funding under the guise of improving the quality of attendant services through language training. There is some tension around this topic, suggesting that not all self-managers like to hire new Canadians as attendants, which partially explains the distinct demographic makeup. Direct Funding does not have straightforward protections against employment discrimination and, in fact, self-managers (and parallel service users in other regions) are encouraged to hire culturally appropriate attendants.

There are many remaining questions in this area, particularly regarding what proportion of attendants are new Canadians, how Independent Living organizations account for the diversity, and how the motivations differ between diverse PSWs in long-term care and the Canadian attendants doing this work while engaged in postsecondary education.

Short-Circuiting Policy Discussions

The rhetorical positioning of attendant services and Direct Funding as "not care" can draw attention away from other policy issues by emphasizing these political messages about disability and care. Yet, the finding that care does not completely disappear under the Direct Funding Program presents a nuanced perspective that is uncommon in the policy realm. This perspective can overwhelm more commonplace policy discussions, such as of worker regulation, and social/health policy divisions.

Struggling to Stay in the Conversation: Regulation of Care Workers

In this study, care is linked to the notion of professionals, with participants ambivalent towards their roles. Care professionals are not welcome to work as attendants under Direct Funding; self-managers are framed as the true experts who are able to train attendants to become specialists in their support. The training under Direct Funding has as much (or perhaps more) to do with conveying Independent Living philosophy as it does with technical, transferable skills. As such, there is resistance to the idea of regulating attendants. Self-manager Isabelle explains:

> I think we're getting away, then, from the whole philosophy of Independent Living. I think regulating, then you're risking unionizing and what you're saying is you have to have certain credentials to do attendant care and it's more institutionalized ... I mean, Direct Funding and Independent Living and directing your own attendants is all about, I think, all about: you hire who you want. It doesn't matter what their credentials are, it's who clicks with you in terms of personality.

"Institutionalized" here does not refer to a physical building but to the abstract sense of a patterned and controlled life. Part of the establishment of the program included securing exceptions under the Regulated Health Professions Act that, as initially proposed, would make services classified as "controlled acts" illegal offences if performed by an uncertified professional; many of the originally proposed controlled acts (e.g., catheterization) are commonly provided by attendants (Yoshida et al. 2004; Roeher Institute 1997). Professionals remain respected for their knowledge and skills regarding specialized medical needs, and at times of crises. As such, care is removed from the Direct Funding context yet not eliminated; rather, care and care professionals are contained to certain contexts.

Contrasting this perspective are a growing number of PSW training programs in Ontario colleges, including several programs offered through private career-training colleges. Further, there have been ongoing public conversations on regulating PSWs and others engaged in similar work (e.g., CBC News 2008, 2011). In 2006, the Health Professions Regulatory Advisory Council advised against the regulation of PSWs but stressed the need for research on PSW educational programs. Following this report, the Ontario Ministry of Health and Long-Term Care created a PSW registry that, though serving an ambiguous role, will eventually be mandatory for all people employed in this type of work. In 2014, the Ontario government released a common education standard for PSWs that replaced three existing standards and seeks to simplify the long-term care sector. Independent Living attendants are lumped into almost all policy discussions of PSWs, though people with disabilities and disability organizations are not always consulted. At other times, attendants are explicitly excluded from policy developments, including initially from the small wage increase for PSWs announced in 2014. Bridging into the developmental service sector, there are efforts to define the core competencies, develop apprenticeship programs, and regulate developmental service workers under Bill 77 (Bill 77 2008). It is noteworthy that people hired under the Ontario Special Services at Home or the Passport programs – individualized funding programs used to assist families of children with physical or developmental disabilities and adults with intellectual disabilities – are even less regulated than those employed under Direct Funding. There is no set wage, no employer requirements, and no mechanisms for mediating disputes.

As in other arenas, the Independent Living perspective presents an unusual narrative in the policy debate. Disability advocates in Ontario have yet to formally come out as being opposed to standardized PSW training and the possibility of worker regulation, and at times serve as consultants, guest speakers, and researchers in college programs and government committees on regulation (e.g., Church, Diamond, and Voronka 2004). With the recent political emphasis on these issues in Ontario and elsewhere in Canada, the Independent Living critique and the benefits associated with the informal, unregulated model may be trampled by a dominating health discourse that includes a preference towards credentialism.

Given reoccurring debates about regulation and the expansion of personal support worker and developmental services worker programs, formalizing the attendant services field in Ontario may be inevitable and could have benefits such as eliminating more questionable programs and false credentials; however,

Independent Living risks being left out of this process. The words of self-managers using the Direct Funding Program challenge the professionalization of attendants in a sophisticated way, but this perspective is underused in these policy discussions. Disability communities in Ontario, however, must clarify their positions on professionalism, as well as their positions on older people, people who cannot "self-direct," and people with more complex health needs – issues that current PSW programs address. Independent Living positioning on this final issue, health, reveals another policy discussion that is short-circuited by the complex position represented by the Direct Funding Program.

A Social Model in a Medical System

Declaring personal support as "not care" under Direct Funding distances it in part from a medical framework and distances disability from illness; indeed, in this study, various health needs are considered appropriate applications of care. As we saw in the previous chapter, theoretically, the line between health and daily needs is clear, but in practice, particularly for the attendants, the distinction can be ambiguous and results in attendants performing tasks beyond their comfort levels.

The shifting boundaries around health have implications beyond the daily interactions, as the Ontario and federal government structures are also divided along health/social lines and the program emerged during a period of health care reform (Yoshida et al. 2004). Ontario's Ministry of Health and Long-Term Care currently funds the Direct Funding Program. Previously, there was a brief period (July 27, 1998–June 17, 1999) during which a separate Ministry of Long-Term Care existed and funded the program. Before that, the Ministry of Community and Social Services (MCSS) funded attendant services, and during the development phase of Direct Funding, much of the background research, political push, and legislative changes required was led by this ministry (Yoshida et al. 2004). MCSS continues to address the needs of people with intellectual disabilities and children with all types of disabilities, and is the government branch responsible for the implementation of the Accessibility for Ontarians with Disabilities Act. This may appear like administrative shuffling; yet, the issue of ministerial placement of Direct Funding was discussed on multiple occasions in this study, particularly by the key informants. Community advocate Andrew says:

> *Andrew:* My ultimate hope is that the Ministry of Health and Long-Term Care will get out of the business of attendant support services ... I

believe that it is a community-based funding model and therefore the Ministry of Community ... of communities?

CK: and Social Services?

Andrew: ... and Social Services has to be involved directly. The Ministry of Health and Long-Term Care deals with patients. It deals with people who are institutionalized in a patient setting. If we want to break the mould of the patient setting, we have to move all the funding and all the programs out of that ministry that deals with attendant support services. And how do you do that? You move it to the ministry that deals with Community and Social Services.

Jennifer, another community advocate, agrees:

CK: So what are some of the current advocacy issues related to attendant care generally, or Direct Funding specifically?

Jennifer: I guess the first is to position it not as care but as a service. From my perspective, that's a mindset that people need to understand. So if it's under Health and Long-Term Care, it automatically gets considered care.

The program aims to not only address a need for attendant services but also to convey a strong cultural message about care, disability, and independence. The key informants, with one exception, expressed that attendant services should not be funded through the health system. Some also felt uncomfortable with the welfare undertones of the MCSS, suggesting other ministries and options.

The restructuring of programs, ministries, and funding in the 1990s was not only administrative reorganizing; it was also connected to the considerable change in the amount and method of federal transfer payments to the provinces. The Canada Assistance Plan was transformed into the smaller Canada Health and Social Transfer in part to help balance the budget, but this switch created a difficult environment for social approaches to health to survive in (McIntosh 2004). The subsequent split into the Canada Health Transfer and the Canada Social Transfer (yet another example of the health/social split in government organization) cemented the priority of providing funding to initiatives linked to health care. With the advent of the Canada Health and Social Transfer in 1996, and even more so with the creation of the Canada Health Transfer and the Canada Social Transfer systems in 2004, more funding, in both cash and tax credits, became available for health-related services. The preference for funding health over social services was bolstered by widespread public and political support, thanks to the almost iconic status of the Canadian health care system (Mahon 2008; see also Armstrong 2001). Community care and attendant services in particular were not adequately addressed by the Romanow commission and its resulting report, a centrepiece of the reform (Shapiro 2003), suggesting further ambiguity as to whether they should be considered health or social services. The political messages that Direct Funding is "not care" fade into the background in light of the long waiting list, insufficient attendant-service hours for many self-managers, and calls for higher wages for attendants, as there is simply more money available for health in Canada. It is thus pragmatic for Independent Living to endorse a health care model at times to gain access to funding increases and address the needs of self-managers on the program.

Concessions must be made to the medical model in order to access funding from the health system. Until 2012, the program managed to sidestep the push to centralize and regionalize many health services through Local Health Integration Networks (LHINs), introduced in 2005 (Ronson 2006). Centralizing health services aims to reduce costs and streamline access but also limits the mobility feature of health care. Direct Funding has a provincial jurisdiction, making it an anomaly that pushes against the localization of services. In 2012, the LHIN system adopted the lead LHIN model in order to devolve provincial programs, like Direct Funding, from the ministry (CILT 2012). During the integration, the Direct Funding Program secured a formal commitment from the ministry that the program could continue to operate under the Independent Living philosophy (CILT 2012). Indeed, insisting on critically, culturally informed messaging of this program led to tangible changes in the health policy realm.

The placement of the program, whether viewed as fiscally strategic or ideologically problematic, has unintended community consequences. Unfortunately, funding the program through the Ontario Ministry of Health and Long-Term Care reinforces community divides between people with physical disabilities and people with intellectual disabilities, and their related organizations and allies, as discussed in the third bridge of accessible care. Even if the political and community will was present to expand the program to include people with intellectual disabilities, the ministerial separation of physical and intellectual disabilities further reduces the likelihood of this happening. The people most affected by this divide are those who have both physical and intellectual disabilities, and who are left to awkwardly bridge multiple systems and occupy diminishing policy spaces. As Jackie, a community advocate and mother of a son with profound physical and intellectual disabilities, describes:

People with developmental disabilities were kind of shunned over in one direction because a lot of the people with physical disabilities felt that it coloured their image in the world, because people might think that people with physical disabilities also had developmental disabilities. They weren't able to distinguish that just because a person has a physical disability doesn't always mean they have a developmental disability. It made it hard for people like [my son] to get what he needed in the physical disability world because he always kept getting shunted into the developmental disability world. We were jumping on both sides of the fence.

The tension between attendant services as "not care" and health needs as care offers the opportunity for a valuable critique of the medical system but highlights the need for more clarification within the community. The ambiguity places attendant services on the edges of funding discussions, since they do not fit neatly in either a health or a social framework.

Closing Thoughts

The seemingly isolated process of distinguishing what care is and is not under Ontario's Direct Funding Program has, in fact, broad policy implications. Generally, this process funnels attention in certain directions, sometimes to the benefit of self-managers, attendants, and Independent Living; at other times, it unintentionally obscures certain policy issues.

Several outcomes arise from the areas that are "not care" – "arms and legs" operations, mandatory relational work, and the relational ontologies between attendants and self-managers. The "arms and legs" descriptor situates attendants as assistive devices and is similar in approach to accessibility legislation, such as the Accessibility for Ontarians with Disabilities Act. This process unfortunately takes the actual provision of the services out of the purview of the various stakeholders, and off the table during vibrant negotiations and discussions of how to implement this legislation. Indeed, by considering attendants as "arms and legs," the focus is on how to make space for the extra limbs, and not on how to ensure the initial presence of the limbs. Relational work is integral to the daily operations of Direct Funding; yet, classifying this work as "not care" and limiting discussions of this aspect of the work in lieu of employer-employee language obscures the ways in which relationships serve to fill in the gaps of the program. The informal, relational ontologies developed in Direct Funding arrangements contribute to the sense that working as an attendant is "not like work," and thus expectations of working conditions do not seem to apply.

Attendants surprisingly do not complain much about the pay, lack of benefits, or short shifts, perhaps because of the student demographic attracted to this line of work and the highly valued relationships that form.

There are also links in the areas that remain care. By linking professionals and care, Independent Living perspectives risk exclusion from discussions related to the education of personal support workers in Ontario, since they could be considered as "having nothing to do with you." The link between care and health and efforts to distance Independent Living from health affected funding and ministry placement. The ambiguity of where Direct Funding fits in unfortunately moves it to the edges of these important discussions. There are many areas of need within the Direct Funding Program, forcing administrators and advocates to concede to the fiscal and cultural reality that more funding opportunities and public support are linked to the health care system than to social services, especially in a period of austerity.

The Direct Funding Program thus plays a complex role within the Ontario policy landscape, despite its relatively small size and scope. Primarily, it works with, rather than against, the precarious economic landscape (Vosko 2000) by drawing on workers who prefer the flexibility and informality of attendant work. There are preliminary indications in this study that Direct Funding may also be cultivating a new demographic of care worker. In comparison with the typical profile of care workers, the attendants in this study are younger and attending postsecondary education, doing this type of work temporarily en route to becoming care professionals of various types. There was also less ethnic diversity and more balance between the sexes in terms of numbers. The Direct Funding Program does not resist the neoliberal economy and models of work, but uses these trends to benefit the program.

The Direct Funding Program retains cultural messages that challenge common understandings of disability and care, and such messages are not often found in government-funded policies and programs. The cultural role is both a detriment and a benefit to the functioning of the program, as it can distance the program from some policy discussions but makes it stand out as a program that is not serving merely a material need but also an ideological one. The messages about disability and care occur alongside neoliberal and austerity rationales. In this particular instance, neoliberal frameworks help justify and sustain the specific program, yet neoliberal policy ideologies notoriously co-opt and undermine the efforts of the nonprofit sector and systematically aim to limit advocacy from this sector. It may be that this mobilizing neoliberal rationale was more effective in justifying the program than was the rights-based social movement messaging about care, as all three major political parties in Ontario supported the program during the early years. It is unlikely that the government and political figures supported, approved, and funded a new program because of compelling disability messaging; rather, the rhetoric of independence, cost-saving, and individual responsibility resonated with their political agendas. In the next chapter, I explore these final issues by examining the implications of linking an organization with a social movement history and network so directly with government administration.

6

Governing Independent Living

Much of Canadian disability organizing has taken place through the creation and maintenance of formally recognized organizations, including those that are registered as charities and nonprofit organizations (Neufeldt 2003). Some of these organizations have long and convoluted histories, given shifts in cultural views and understandings of disability, resulting in sometimes contradictory positions on disability over time (Carey and Gu 2014). Social movement scholars comment on the process whereby grassroots organizing evolves (sometimes in order to survive) into professionalized and formalized organizations, a process that may or may not replace the original activities (M. Smith 2005; Young and Everitt 2004; Phillips 1999; Carroll 1997). Establishing a social movement organization with explicit social justice aims, or even simply a nonprofit organization, includes building a strong membership base; determining core activities and services; acquiring physical space; seeking formal recognition through nonprofit or charitable status; developing revenue streams; adopting business structures such as a board of directors; and hiring management and staff.

Creating nonprofit organizations may be an essential step in establishing the voice of a group and ensuring longevity of a social movement, and formalizing these organizations has many advantages. However, the increasing professionalization of social movement organizations also has detrimental consequences, as explored in a collection of articles on the status of social movement organizing in the United States titled *The Revolution Will Not Be Funded: Beyond the Non-Profit Industrial Complex* (Incite! Women of Color against Violence 2007). The collection pays particular attention to the role of large and small foundation-granting agencies within the US nonprofit sector, with echoes of the Canadian reliance on government funding and its attendant issues (Levasseur 2012). Andrea Smith (2007, 10), in her introduction to the collection, explains:

> NPIC [the nonprofit industrial complex] contributes to a mode of organizing that is ultimately unsustainable. To radically change society, we must build mass movements that can topple systems of domination, such as capitalism. However, the NPIC encourages us to think of social justice organizing as a career; that is, you do the work if you can get paid for it.

She further adds, "The NPIC promotes a social movement culture that is non-collaborative, narrowly focused and competitive" (10). Indeed, the professionalization of a social movement often requires compromising radical goals and diluting movement messages in ways that will appease funding sources and directly or indirectly divide communities. In relation to disability, these issues are further complicated by ambiguity as to which organizations can or should be considered part of a larger social movement, as many disability-related organizations operate in whole or in part within charitable or medical frameworks.

CILT's administration of the government-funded Direct Funding Program also has consequences for the Canadian Independent Living movement. The Canadian Independent Living network grapples with identifying as a social movement, perhaps as a survival tactic amid a harsh neoliberal and austerity context. The cultural critiques of care and the political tactics of the Independent Living movement become frozen by program administration, which requires clear and consistent messaging. This leads to both individual and collective fear of losing funding and, significantly, diverges from policy approaches emerging from other elements of disability organizing and communities in Ontario. Although Direct Funding fits among numerous policy trends, it is incongruous with the transformation of the developmental service sector, as well as with developments encompassed by the UN Convention on the Rights of Persons with Disabilities, and may entrench long-standing divides among impairment groups in Ontario. Outside the policy realm, the removal of care from attendant services and the administrative role of Independent Living centres do not align with the approaches of an emerging generation of disability activists, as demonstrated by new leaders and approaches featured at a 2011 Youth Activist Forum in Ottawa, Doing Disability Differently, and globally represented by those doing disability justice work or radical disability politics in the wake of austerity.

Nonprofit Organizations under Neoliberal Governance

In the wake of neoliberalism and the advent of austerity policy frameworks, the governments' roles shift to regulate the workforce (e.g., for PSW workers, the Transformation initiative related to the developmental service sector), monitor the public and private sectors (e.g., the AODA and the UN convention), and administer funds for external agencies to provide services (e.g., the Direct Funding Program). Neoliberalism is characterized by, among other traits, changing relationships between governments and the nonprofit sector. In Canadian contexts, this includes the shift from core-funding arrangements for nonprofit organizations to project-based competitions that include service delivery. The Canadian nonprofit sector historically relies heavily on funding from government sources, and disability-related organizations are no exception (Hall and Banting 2000). Levesque (2012) investigated the human, financial, and technological capacity of fifteen Canadian disability organizations and found that the lack of core operating funds greatly diminished the organizations' ability to offer innovative programming, gesturing towards the barriers facing disability organizations within a hostile sociopolitical climate. The core activities and agendas of nonprofit organizations are shaped by eligibility criteria and program priorities linked to these changing opportunities.

Many nonprofit organizations have social movement histories, which means that government agencies and departments play unusually strong roles in determining the priorities of leading Canadian social movement organizations by setting guidelines and administering project-based funding. Federal and provincial funding programs often include lengthy application and reporting requirements, mobilized though the rhetoric of transparency and accountability (Hall and Banting 2000). As such, organizations that successfully obtain funding can end up dedicating a disproportionate amount of time and resources to managing these funds, to the detriment of other work. Canadian nonprofit organizations find themselves in a funding conundrum in which they are reliant on the funding competitions but largely immobilized by the administrative requirements. This Canadian funding conundrum contrasts with the situation of social movement organizations that engage in direct action *against* governments – for example, the disability group ADAPT in the United States (*ADAPT Free Our People!* 2010). American organizations do face similar issues with other powerful groups because of the reliance on charitable foundations.

Nonprofit organizations with a social justice component or history in particular must turn away from activist work that is "un-fundable" for lack of measurable, short-term outputs (M. Smith 2005). Various levels of government become "objective" regulators, evaluating the very services they underfund. The evaluations are often further outsourced to independent consultants, sometimes from within the communities governments seek to monitor and regulate – for example, the Roeher Institute (affiliated with the Canadian Association for Community Living), which evaluated the pilot version of the Direct Funding Program (Roeher Institute 1997). These are early observations on the relationship between nonprofit organizations and Canadian governments, and the course may change. The consequences, however, for the Independent Living movement and disability movements are less tentative.

Independent Living as a Social Movement

In this shifting environment, the Direct Funding Program stands remarkably still. In many ways, Direct Funding is the quintessential manifestation of Independent Living philosophy as it was originally conceived; it embodies many of the philosophical tenets identified by John Lord (2010), including consumer control, cross-disability (to an extent, in that it is not only for people with a certain impairment), peer-support, integration, and full participation, and functioning as a nonprofit organization. Writing in the United Kingdom, Jenny Morris (1993, 17) identifies central tenets of a broader Independent Living movement:

1. All human life is of value.
2. Anyone, whatever their impairment, is capable of exerting choices.
3. People who are disabled by society have a right to assert control over their lives.
4. Disabled people have the right to participate fully in society.

The tenets of cross-disability and "whatever their impairments" do not entirely fit with the Direct Funding Program, but the emphasis on self-determination, consumer control, community integration, and participation are defining characteristics of the program and can be easily located in public materials produced by CILT. For example, CILT's website describes Independent Living as a "vision, a philosophy and a movement of persons with disabilities," and outlines a philosophy with tenets similar to those cited above.

A tension exists between the history and philosophy of Independent Living as a social movement and the willingness of Canadian Independent Living organizations to publicly identify as an activist or advocacy network. It is generally agreed that Canadian Independent Living has strong activist roots and should be considered a movement, as stated on CILT's website (Lord 2010;

Hutchison, Arai, Pedlar, Lord, and Yuen 2007; Valentine 1994). Further, in addition to the key informants approached in this study for their involvement in community activism, many of the self-managers and informal supports, and even a few of the attendants, reported engaging in various individual advocacy efforts and collective actions. The participants described times when they pushed against schools, businesses, governments, and workplaces for inclusion of disabled people. Yet, Independent Living centres avoid engaging in activism or advocacy in a formal capacity. As CILT's (CILT 2010) website explains, "Independent Living Resource Centres do not engage in collective advocacy. Instead, the Independent Living movement promotes an end to institutional living for people with disabilities and encourages and supports individuals to integrate into the community." This is partly because of charitable status, which in Canada cannot be assigned to organizations with political purposes, including efforts to "retain, oppose, or change the law, policy, or decision of any level of government in Canada or a foreign country" (Canada Revenue Agency 2011). Securing funding without charitable status is very difficult; thus, applying for this status is an appealing route for nonprofit organizations.

The aversion to activism is also partly connected to the history of Independent Living in Canada. Lord (2010, 159) notes that "the Canadian Independent Living movement decided early on that it would stress individual advocacy (and self-advocacy), not collective advocacy. In part, this decision was made because [the Council of Canadians with Disabilities] and other national groups were already doing the collective advocacy." The distinction between individual, self, and collective advocacy may not be as clear as Lord implies, since the self-advocacy focus creates a tension with the notion of Independent Living as a collective movement. Even the example of the messages rejecting care documented in this study could be considered a form of cultural activism, though the Direct Funding example lends itself to stagnation because the messages are necessarily frozen, enshrined as they are in binding policy documents and eligibility criteria. Regardless of the rationale, Independent Living centres and the national Independent Living office tend to publicly promote self-advocacy, systems navigation, and life skills, rather than collective action.

Based on academic accounts of Canadian disability movements, as well as on the philosophical tenets listed above, the Direct Funding Program in many ways *is* Independent Living in Ontario. It emerged through advocacy and activism, but no confrontational tactics were used (or at least were not documented), a feature that distinguishes Canadian disability movements from American ones, according to Chivers (2007) and Barnartt (2008). It is situated in the nonprofit sector and would fit into the histories of disability advocacy outlined by Neufeldt (2003). It represents an ongoing relationship with the Ontario government, as many politicians and public servants are identified as allies, not adversaries, in the history, among other accomplishments (Prince 2012; Peters 2003; Stienstra 2003; Valentine 1996; Valentine and Vickers 1996). Joel, an executive employee at one of the Ontario Independent Living centres, explains how Direct Funding is the showpiece program, the one highlighted in requests for elusive, core funding:

> We're developing a case for support [for core funding] and in there we've made a case in terms of how we align to a lot of what the government of Ontario is doing. We profile the Direct Funding Program as one of the most concrete examples of Independent Living. So it's important to the movement, for sure.

As mentioned, Direct Funding is in many ways philosophically representative of the Independent Living approach and operationally reflective of the documented Canadian disability movements. It may create a conflict of interest for Canadian social movements to receive core funding from governments when advocacy often takes the form of policy formation and consultation.

Independent Living in Canada and CILT are clear examples of social movement organizations adapting and responding to a hostile sociopolitical climate (M. Smith 2005). Nonprofit certification and the obtaining of charitable status are essential survival strategies in the present context, with several unanticipated implications. These implications include tendencies to distance from activist language in public materials in order to broaden funding options, which raises questions about the evolving roles of nonprofit organizations with social movement histories. There are remnants and occasional examples of "empowerment" and other social justice language in these organizations, and even in the government-funded programs. Yet, accountability to government requires an uncomfortable administration of empowerment in ways that can be documented, measured, and reported. In an austerity climate, disability organizations are often forced into service delivery under a continual threat of extinction. The organizations may manage to incorporate social justice messaging when possible, but it is unclear if these messages further the cause of disability justice in substantial ways.

Care as Oppression and Fears of Losing Funding
Like many other social movements, the Canadian Independent Living movement has developed a network of nonprofit organizations, and this formalization

affects the broader messages of disability activism in Canada. One of the clearest outcomes can be seen in how the messages about care in the Direct Funding Program diverge from other approaches to disability as well as in individual self-managers and Independent Living organizations, both of whom demonstrate a strong fear of losing gains brought about by dependency on government funding.

Self-managers expressed a strong fear of losing their direct funding; this is likely linked to their aversion to other available attendant-service options and the enduring legacies of oppressive forms of care. Direct-funding styles of attendant services are broadly associated with high levels of user satisfaction, increased sense of control and empowerment, and more flexibility and freedom than with other arrangements (e.g., Blyth and Gardner 2007; Caldwell and Heller 2007; Stainton and Boyce 2004; Williams et al. 2003; Parker et al. 2000; Roeher Institute 1997). In this study, self-managers expressed their satisfaction with the Direct Funding Program, particularly when compared with other attendant arrangements. Eighteen out of twenty self-managers used at least one other type of attendant services before receiving direct funding, and ten of them used two or more types of attendant services before Direct Funding. The self-managers unanimously preferred the Direct Funding model over the past arrangements for various reasons, including choice of attendants, flexibility, and control over schedule. However, these results, as well as those of the studies noted above, do not consider the satisfaction of people on the Direct Funding waiting list, those ineligible to apply to the program, or those who have been rejected by the program.

The satisfaction of self-managers in this study is linked to personal histories of more oppressive attendant-service arrangements, including abuse, thus demonstrating the tensions of care. One self-manager approached to participate in this study declined precisely because of a fear of losing his funding. Near the end of our interview, self-manager Jason candidly says:

I always had a feeling that deep down, if I'm going to be totally honest with myself and honest with you, it's always been a bit of fear for me of Direct Funding, that is, like keep your head down. Don't ruffle, don't rock the boat ... Try to fly under the radar. It's good to be under the radar because they will take your funding away if you're in the radar. And there was a real fear for me that if I ever have a problem with one of my [attendants], a situation that I don't know how to deal with, the last person I'm gonna call is Direct Funding ... But my big deep dark secret fear is that they're gonna see that as weakness, that you're not able to deal with the funding. And say, oh, you don't know how to handle that situation, well, you shouldn't be directing your own funding.

The personal histories of more oppressive arrangements, combined with satisfaction with Direct Funding, confirm that self-managers have a lot to lose. Losing their funding would mean going back to a less than ideal living arrangement, one with more of a caring (oppressive in this instance) approach to disability, less control and flexibility, and perhaps a higher risk of abuse. This fear also shows the gains of Independent Living are constrained by funding accountability networks.

The fear of losing funding can also be seen on an institutional level in the materials and Direct Funding interview process facilitated through the Centre for Independent Living in Toronto. For example, the *Financial Administration Start-Up Package for Self-Managers and Bookkeepers* (CILT 2008), a publication given to all approved self-managers, details the complicated financial reporting requirements, yet it ultimately recommends that self-managers hire bookkeepers and a payroll service. It contains strong disciplinary language, with many directives – for example, sentences beginning with "You must" and "You need" – along with repeated reminders of the consequences of the "failure" to manage the funds properly. Reading the publication, one feels overwhelmed by the complex and rigid requirements. There were many challenges in initially securing approval for the Direct Funding Program (Yoshida et al. 2004); it is likely that CILT's documents reflect the organization's concerns about losing this hard-won funding, which is integral to the strength of CILT and to keeping other Independent Living centres afloat in Ontario. The political landscape makes these more individualized forms of service delivery probable in the future, but this must be balanced with the consistent underfunding of nonprofit organizations, particularly those linked to social movements. CILT exists in a tenuous context, where core funding is almost nonexistent and organizations are highly dependent on project-based opportunities and service delivery programs, such as the Direct Funding Program. CILT, just like the self-managers, has a lot to lose in terms of Direct Funding.

The Direct Funding qualification interviews are extolled as different from professional evaluations at other attendant programs since they are conducted by a board of peers (people with disabilities, often self-managers); however, they may in fact contribute to the fear of losing funding. Self-manager Marc recounts:

If I have a job interview and I fail at a job interview, then there's going to be another job interview. But if I failed at the Direct Funding [interview], then I can't live in my house. I can't continue with my job. You know, my entire life would have changed. So I had to pass this interview. And since it was the first time that I ever did something like that, I didn't know how strict they were, I didn't know what the criteria were, I didn't know. You know, it's the first time, I had no details about it, so I was extremely stressed for that interview.

The intense application and interview process is designed to determine if the potential applicant has the skills required to legally act as an employer. The final evaluation of the pilot project makes ambiguous references to a "standardize[d] assessment of self-management skills" developed by CILT that potential self-managers are scored on during the interview (Roeher Institute 1997, 32). The model is committed to accommodation, inclusion, and consumer control; as such, it is concerning that CILT does not publicly publish the criteria for the assessment and, further, that people are evaluated and scored (presumably) on their intelligence and learning skills within a cross-disability organization. One couple spoke in detail about the preparation they felt was necessary for their Direct Funding interview, including making "thirteen pages of cheat notes." The potential self-managers were particularly concerned about being able to recall relevant employment legislation, vacation pay rules, and so on, during the interview. The fear is both individual and institutional, and reflective of the shifting landscape and changing relationships between Canadian nonprofit organizations and governments.

Framing care as oppressive can be tied to a fear of losing funding, since other arrangements are depicted and reported as being less empowering; however, this detracts from an important exclusion embedded in the program's eligibility requirements. The ability to self-direct is emphasized throughout CILT's material on Direct Funding, but it's an ability that diminishes as one ages. Perhaps the tone of urgency and the emphasis on self-direction in the documents are unnecessarily amplified; other direct-funding programs, notably in the United Kingdom, operate differently. The United Kingdom is seeing a push from governments as well as from the disability community to get *more* people on Direct Payments (C. Barnes 2007), using whatever supports are needed to make this feasible. The emphasis for the UK model is not on reporting, accountability, and self-direction, but on solutions that make Direct Payments suitable for various individuals (Ridley and Jones 2003; Leece 2000;

Maglajlic, Brandon, and Given 2000). This is but one example, within a larger trend, of where Independent Living and the messages enshrined in the Direct Funding Program diverge from approaches to intellectual disability.

Diverging from Approaches to Intellectual Disability

Support for people with intellectual disabilities, which can include support with decision making, is still considered a form of care by some study participants. The final evaluation report of the pilot project, written by the Roeher Institute in the mid-1990s, notes:

> "Self-management capacity" as defined for the purposes of this Project might unnecessarily exclude individuals who may need assistance in self-management because of a lack of management skills or because of a deteriorating condition. Self-management, at least in theory, does not appear to be at odds with a recognition of the need for support. (Roeher Institute 1997, iii)

The exclusion of people with intellectual disabilities from the Direct Funding Program stood out in the early days of the program and was solidified by the movement of attendant services from the Ministry of Community and Social Services (where most services for people with intellectual disabilities continue to reside) to the Ministry of Health and Long-Term Care. Direct Funding departs from other developments in the disability field, as further demonstrated through the provincial transformation of the developmental service sector and the UN Convention on the Rights of Persons with Disabilities.

The Transformation initiative in Ontario, situated in the Ministry of Community and Social Services, alongside but peculiarly separate from efforts regarding the AODA, began in 2004 and included closing the doors of the last large-scale institutions in the province in March 2009 (Community Living Ontario 2009). Deinstitutionalization in Ontario was heralded by the disability community, especially people with intellectual disabilities and their allies (Community Living Ontario 2009; Stroman 2003). Through this historic process it became apparent that existing legislation was outdated: it assumed institutionalization as the preferred response to disability and employed language considered offensive by contemporary standards. Thus, it was necessary to "transform" the legislation and practices of the Ontario developmental service sector.

A significant portion of the Transformation initiative and related Bill 77 builds on past advocacy of the Special Services at Home (SSAH) program (SSAH Provincial Coalition 2011) and the work of the Individualized Funding Coalition for Ontario (2008) proposing to expand individualized funding to support people with intellectual disabilities. A dynamic relationship exists between the Direct Funding Program and individualized funding, as SSAH served as a precedent when establishing Direct Funding, and Direct Funding served as a model to support requests for more substantive individualized approaches for people with developmental disabilities. Through the Transformation initiative, SSAH has been expanded and a new version, titled Passport, was introduced specifically for adults eighteen years or older and who have developmental disabilities. Unlike Direct Funding, the money can be used for an array of purposes related to living with an intellectual disability, and the emphasis is not on personal care needs. For example, Martha, a parent advocate, explains what her family used SSAH for:

> Because it was individualized funding, we could be flexible with it, so we developed – I had to think back to my days as a civil service manager, how do you structure a budget? You ballpark it, and then you don't have to stick to that as long as you can explain how you diverged. So we put in a certain amount for the staffing, and we wanted to pay those people well once we got them. There was some money; it could go for training them, it could go for [my son] to go somewhere with them to hear a presentation about [a] meaningful day or whatever, it went for mileage for our vehicle ... His YMCA membership came from the budget, his rental of his assisted devices computer because they wouldn't pay it 100 percent – they paid for wheelchairs 100 percent but they wouldn't pay for devices, so that went in there.

Similarly, community researcher Thomas describes how individualized funding works for his family and in the bigger picture:

> So, for example, if I think about my own daughter, who is thirty now, and she has a couple of pockets of individualized funding, she has Special Services at Home, she also has Passport funding. She's living with a friend in a house. For her to really manage that money and use it effectively requires some facilitation support, it requires somebody to spend time with her, help her figure stuff out, spend time with her figuring [out] who she's gonna hire, when and how, how to follow up on her dreams. I think the assumption in

the Independent Living movement is that the person can do it themselves, can do all those things. The assumption in the individualized funding movement, where it's more family-driven and more around people with developmental disabilities, the assumption is more that people are going to need some facilitation support to go with that.

Promoting individualized funding options is a substantial part of the Transformation process, and requirements to independently self-direct are conspicuously absent. Ironically, people with physical disabilities will be excluded from accessing any funding resulting from the transformation, which may actually end up requiring less administrative work and providing more flexibility than the Direct Funding Program.[1] In the early days of Direct Funding, there was an unwillingness to complicate the model by including people with intellectual disabilities and others who cannot self-direct. It is unlikely that direct and individualized funding options will unify in the future, in part because of the ministerial separation of services for people with physical disabilities and those with intellectual disabilities. The Transformation initiative demonstrates an alternative way to administer individualized funding in a Canadian context, and Ontario's Direct Funding Program may be unnecessarily rigid when it comes to the requirement for an individual to demonstrate the ability to self-direct.

The second example where Direct Funding departs from approaches to intellectual disability is in the context of the UN Convention on the Rights of Persons with Disabilities. The convention was adopted by the UN General Assembly in December 2006 and opened for signature in March 2007, with Canada being one of the first countries to sign it (Foreign Affairs and International Trade Canada 2009). The central aim of the convention is to "protect the right to equality and non-discrimination for persons with disabilities," which branches into issues of reasonable accommodation (MacQuarrie 2010). It is acclaimed as the fastest negotiated international convention, and Canadians played a substantial role in this negotiation, in particular through the work both the Council of Canadians with Disabilities and the Canadian Association for Community Living. As of December 2014, the convention had 159 signatories and 151 ratifications (United

---

[1] It is beyond the scope of this book to fully investigate the Special Services at Home and Passport funding programs, but there are indications that these programs have led to long waiting lists and confusion, and threaten the survival of many service organizations that rely on transfer payments for past service delivery (since funding is being streamed directly to the individual).

Nations Enable 2014). Many of the ratifications include reservations and interpretative declarations, and in the Canadian example, the federal government has an interpretive declaration on Article 33, item 2, to clarify that monitoring of the convention will account for Canada's federated structure. More significantly, the government put forth a limited reservation and interpretative declarations on three items under Article 12.

In essence, by declaring that people with disabilities shall "enjoy legal capacity on an equal basis with others in all aspects of life" (12(2)) and be supported to do so (12(3)), Article 12 codifies an interdependent understanding of personhood and autonomy that is distinctly different from the definitions of independence operating in the Direct Funding Program. It is not coincidental that the Canadian Association for Community Living has expertise in the area of legal decision making, recognized both nationally and internationally for the model known as "supported decision making," a model reflected throughout Article 12. The supported decision-making model recognizes that all people make decisions with consideration for and with the help of other people, and thus people with intellectual disabilities should not be dismissed as entirely incapable of making complex decisions (Bach and Rock 1996). The supported decision-making model "presumes capacity" and refuses to categorize any individuals as subhuman (Bach and Rock 1996, 6). This approach resonates with the philosophical work as seen in Eva Feder Kittay and Licia Carlson's edited collection *Cognitive Disability and Its Challenge to Moral Philosophy*, in which various authors passionately assert new forms of personhood and methods for enabling participation of those with different ways of being in the world (Kittay and Carlson 2010).

Article 12 acknowledges how experiences and expressions of autonomy for all people rely on caring relationships (Clement 1996). More concretely, it presents a challenge to substitute decision-making models such as power of attorney and guardianship typically employed in legal settings, including in Canada. As written, Article 12 requires a substantial revision of the legal system, and could be interpreted to require the elimination of small- and large-scale institutions that often preclude the conditions for substitute decision making, and challenges the foundational social values of independence and self-determination. Michael Bach, executive vice-president of the Canadian Association for Community Living, writes:

Along with many other people with disabilities, there is a large group of people with more significant intellectual disabilities whose legal capacity, and therefore full personhood before the law[,] is questioned and often removed only because of their ascribed disability status. Article 12 of the convention demands an end to this systemic discrimination. (Bach 2009, n.p.)

This innovative approach seems to directly challenge that of Independent Living and the values behind Direct Funding, which emphasizes independent self-management. For example, the publication *Direct Funding General Information* could be interpreted as questioning the full personhood of people with intellectual disabilities:

> In addition to the ability to self-direct, they must be able to self-manage. A self-manager is a person in control of his or her own situation and not easily manipulated. A self-manager is a person who knows what services he or she wants and needs, someone with plans – perhaps to move, work or study – or simply a clear desire to take responsibility for improving his or her own services. Self-managers are capable of interviewing, training, hiring and if necessary, firing attendants, and handling the financial and reporting duties of an employer. They are willing to take risks in return for the choice, flexibility and control over their attendant services made possible under [Direct Funding]. (CILT 2000, 2)

This passage implies that most people with intellectual disabilities or who require support with the tasks described cannot be considered self-managers. The UN convention endorses a nuanced perspective that aims to enable inclusion for people with an array of capabilities, whereas Direct Funding is designed to work only under certain conditions, for certain individuals.

These two arenas, the provincial Transformation initiative and the UN convention, indicate that rejecting care through the Direct Funding Program and reserving it for people with intellectual disabilities may end up leaving Independent Living and people with physical disabilities behind or on separate paths from people with intellectual disabilities, as reflected in the third bridge of accessible care. Indeed, these two processes perhaps represent future policy approaches to disability, and yet seem separate from the AODA (though, arguably, has more links to the physical disability world), Independent Living, and the once cutting-edge Direct Funding Program.

Disability Activism Outside Policy Spheres and the Nonprofit Sector

Other branches of Canadian disability movements are less documented and discussed than are Independent Living, Community Living, and the realm of public policy; another project I was involved with while researching for this book demonstrated this. From 2006 to 2013, I was a volunteer board member for Citizens with Disabilities – Ontario (CWDO) and a full member of the Council of Canadians with Disabilities (CWDO 2011). In partnership with the Council of Canadians with Disabilities, a group of us fundraised and organized a Youth Activist Forum for approximately forty youth with and without disabilities, held June 3–5, 2011, in Ottawa. As will be seen shortly, it is noteworthy that Independent Living Canada declined to partner on this project. We brought youth together so they might learn from established and emerging leaders with disabilities, and we encouraged the participation of allies in order to position people with disabilities as leaders for all. This was also a participatory action research project funded by the Canadian Centre on Disability Studies (Kelly and Carson 2012). CWDO exists almost exclusively online and does not yet have charitable status. Our lack of resources and infrastructure leaves room for varied projects to emerge, as long as there is a committed leader or group available to volunteer the time. We faced many of the same contextual barriers when planning this event as Independent Living centres do, including confronting the project-based funding landscape and the aversion to including activism in funding proposals (see Kelly and Carson 2012).

Canadian scholars are concerned about a lack of new disability leaders coming to the fore of Independent Living in Canada (Lord 2010; Prince 2009; Hutchison, Arai, Pedlar, Lord, and Whyte 2007). The Youth Activist Forum helps show that youth leaders are present and working but do not necessarily work within the Independent Living model. The forum featured people like jes sachse, an Ontario artist with a disability who is best known for their large-scale, culture-jamming ad campaign American Able done in collaboration with photographer Holly Norris. The campaign spoofs the company American Apparel, a "socially aware company" that, despite its highly sexualized advertising, claims to represent everyday women – yet does not feature women with disabilities (Norris 2011). Sachse's work is known for its commentary not only on disability but also on sexuality, gender, and normalcy. Similarly, sprOUT, a group made up of youth with intellectual disabilities from the Griffin Centre Mental Health Services in Toronto and who identify as gay, lesbian, bisexual, transgendered, or questioning, was invited to present its documentary Our Compass (see Art Gallery of Ontario 2011). By openly sharing their overlapping and shifting identities, sprOUT members represent a highly intersectional approach to disability politics. We featured Jeff Preston, a community activist who independently organized the Mobilize March (Preston 2008) to protest the lack of local accessible transportation, then made a documentary about it, and who is also the writer for the political webcomic *Cripz* (Madrenas and Preston 2011). Preston also spearheads a "stair bombing" initiative, where staircases are humorously closed with yellow caution tape – indeed a confrontational approach to addressing inaccessible built environments (Preston 2011). There are many other examples from these individuals and others (see Kelly 2013). These creative youth leaders are overlooked by and distinct from the Independent Living movement and the approach to disability enshrined in the Direct Funding Program, and this raises questions about whether there is room for individual, intersectional, radical, culturally focused activism within the formally documented and recognized Canadian disability movements.

In 2010, Independent Living Canada and John Lord released a book on the history of Independent Living in Canada. Lord (2010, 35 and 55) comments: "The initial principles of the Independent Living movement are as relevant today as they were in the early 1980s. This in itself is quite remarkable considering that the movement has matured in some significant ways over the last 25 years." "The core functions," he continues, "have changed slightly over the years, but the heart of the original four remain within all centres across Canada." In particular, the Direct Funding Program has seen very few changes to the eligibility criteria, application package, number of recipients, and informational material since it was established as a full-fledged program in 1998. In 2014, the program received an increase in funding that will enable approximately three hundred more people with disabilities to become self-managers and included a slight increase in the maximum number of hours, yet the eligibility criteria remained the same. Even the key informants identified by the centres are many of the same people involved in the program's formation. Is the stability of the Independent Living approach in Canada laudable, or does it represent a fracturing of tactics between emerging and established leaders? Or, is it reflective of organizations trying to remain in operation in a changeable political climate? The consistency may provide stability to CILT, specifically in the current difficult hyper-neoliberal climate, though not necessarily to the Independent Living movement as a whole or other Independent Living centres. The radical arts-based, disability justice, and anti-poverty approaches of the youth leaders is pushed out of Independent Living, highlighted especially by the exclusion of people with intellectual disabilities from Direct Funding – the third, and broken, bridge of accessible care. In the shift from second- to third-wave feminisms, prominent second-wave leaders accused women of a lack of leadership, apathy, and using ineffective political strategies. If we reflect back on the emergence of do-it-yourself feminism in the early 1990s, it is now apparent that the second-wave leaders were misinterpreting the intent and efforts of the new generation (Pinterics 2001; Steenbergen 2001).

The fissures in Canadian disability movement are especially apparent when exploring the example of DAMN (Disability Action Movement Now) 2025. Representatives of this group also attended the 2011 Youth Activist Forum. The Accessibility of Ontarians with Disabilities Act (AODA) aims to make the province of Ontario accessible in all sectors by the year 2025. This policy mechanism was largely supported by disability organizations, and there is a presumption that it is a general good within the Ontario policy landscape. DAMN 2025 speaks back both to the presumed unity of disability advocacy in Ontario and to the specific policy by "damning" long-term promises of inclusion and calling for a more radical and immediate overhaul of the system (DAMN 2025 2008; Henderson 2007). In addition to the radical orientation, DAMN 2025 promotes cross-issue politics and has strong connections with anti-poverty mobilizing in Ontario. DAMN 2025 members have even critiqued the Direct Funding Program; some of these critiques are directed at the Ministry of Health and Long-Term Care; others, at the Centre for Independent Living in Toronto (Anne Abbott, pers. comm.). Unquestionably, Independent Living in Canada and current academic accounts of Canadian disability movements largely overlook these more radical and complex examples of organizing.

The examples from the Youth Activist Forum reflect a broader trend in disability organizing. In the United States, a cross-issue, radical, and transformative approach that moves beyond rights-based and speaks back to Independent Living discourses has been termed "disability justice." Mingus (2011) explains:

> With disability justice, we want to move away from the "myth of independence," that everyone can and should be able to do everything on their own. I am not fighting for independence, as much of the disability rights movement rallies behind. I am fighting for an interdependence that embraces need and tells the truth: no one does it on their own and the myth of independence is just that, a myth.

Beyond this nuanced approach to politics, disabled protesters play a more visible role in mass protests, and the maltreatment of disabled protesters has garnered substantial and muddied media attention. At the G20 protests in Toronto in 2010, John Pruyn reported to the mainstream media that he was "roughed up by police, stripped of his prosthetic leg and detained without charge" (CBC News 2010). In the same year in the United Kingdom, activist Jody McIntyre was pulled out of his wheelchair and dragged by police during student protests against government cuts; this incident was captured on video. Slater (2012, 724) argues, "As a politically active young disabled person, [McIntyre] disturbed the discourses of passivity that surround disability, converging with the demonizing discourses of dangerous youth." In the cases of both Pruyn and McIntyre, extensive media coverage was confused by notions of pity, disapproval of the protests, and concern about whether such "vulnerable" people should exercise their rights to protest. The befuddled media coverage illuminates the ongoing challenges to changing perceptions about disability in cultures that continue to place disability in the realms of medicine and charity. In any case, the tactics and messages deployed by these radical activists are starkly different from those of Independent Living movements ushering in, and in some cases administering, Direct Funding programs throughout the developed world. The Youth Activist Forum, disability justice framework, and Pruyn and McIntyre illustrate a contested field of globalized disability activism, with varied actors, tensions, and complexity that challenge the notion of a singular disability movement in Canada or elsewhere.

Closing Thoughts

Like social movements around the globe, Canadian disability movements are evolving to adapt to shifting contexts and issues. The roles and prominence of organizations, individuals, events, policies, and programs that are cited in historical accounts as "founders" of the movement are changing. Many of the same individuals are still present, but they are forced to adapt to the new environment. This often means seeking funding in the project-based landscape, making concessions to a health model, building on past relationships with governments, and getting into the business of service delivery. Many of the nonprofits behind some of the biggest wins for disability in Canada are struggling to keep afloat in the current context.

I agree with Lord (2010) that the Independent Living movement in Canada has the capacity for social innovation and a proven track record of entrepreneurial spirit. Unfortunately, as seen with the example of the Direct Funding Program, the Independent Living movement is shaped and constrained by the tenuous funding and political environment in Canada. The established relationships with governments may constrain the Independent Living movement from accommodating new leaders and issues, compounding the organizational aversion to activism in spite of the collective history of Independent Living. The programmatic responsibilities of Direct Funding may dilute the cultural messages and roles of Independent Living. This is seen in the concessions to the health model, which do not fit with the strong anti-medical undercurrents of Independent Living philosophy. Freezing program eligibility requirements in ways that exclude people with intellectual disabilities and perpetuate messages that seem out of step with the emerging approaches to intellectual disability further entrenches divides among Ontario disability communities. Finally, failing to acknowledge the diversity of approaches and issues represented by youth leaders in Ontario (while lamenting a lack of youth leadership) will not draw these individuals into leadership roles within the formal Independent Living network.

Youth are engaging in different forms of activism on different issues. Many young leaders with disabilities are involved in cross-issue movements, such as the Quebec student movement, the Occupy movement, and Idle No More. The approach of these leaders is very different from the approaches documented in historical accounts of Canadian disability movements. The approaches are so different that they may be overlooked by the previous generations that comment on the lack of new leadership. Youth leaders and contemporary activism operate more on the level of cultural meaning making – or what Garland-Thomson (2009, 193) calls "visual activism" – than on the level of policy making, and work with and across diverse identities. These youth leaders may find it difficult to frame their work in terms of deliverables and project management, and may perhaps also find that the formal organizations are too restrictive for their work.

The disconnect between the founding generation of Canadian disability activists and the emerging cultural, cross-issue approaches of youth leaders represents both a maturing and a division of the movement. The youth activities make clear that there are many strands of disability organizing in Canada. Yet, the disconnect also reveals a gap wherein the established organizations and leaders are reluctant to incorporate and recognize new approaches, issues, and leaders.

Conclusion
Removing Care Amid a "Crisis of Care"

The provision of care remains a gendered and devalued field of work that is deeply intertwined with oppression. The stubborn devaluation of care is perplexing because people are confronted with the availability of services at points of crisis in their lives, and there is ongoing media and public policy attention to the provision of care for older people. Headlines in mainstream media emphasize issues related to caring for the aging demographic or for people with certain illnesses, such as cancer, more often than for people with disabilities. It is common to read and hear stories documenting worker shortages in long-term care facilities, poor conditions in public facilities, frail older people ending up in emergency rooms after falls and other incidents, inadequate home care support, and strained informal support networks, among other issues. More positive stories cover the promise of technologies that help to monitor older people at home, increase independence, and prevent accidents (e.g., see Calacare 2013). In academic and policy circles, concepts such as aging in place, healthy aging, and age-friendly communities circulate broadly, signifying sustained attention towards and innovation in the questions of care (e.g., Wiles et al. 2012; Plouffe and Kalache 2010; World Health Organization 2007; Peel, Bartlett, and McClure 2004). Addressing the "crisis of care" for the aging population, preferably within home-based settings, is a central issue in Canada and globally.

In Ontario and elsewhere, there is a building sense of urgency to address issues of long-term care, perhaps reflecting what Katz (1992) terms "alarmist demography," where older populations are presented as a neoliberal problem. The "problem" of care for older people is positioned as an impending disaster premised on current service inadequacies; subjects that are easy to discuss but difficult to resolve. Unlike this widespread and at times alarmist attention to care for older people, attendant services remain in what Titchkosky (2011) calls the "not yet" time of disability. Titchkosky (2011, 108) explains, "One dominant conception is that disability is a category of partial inclusion steeped in an ambiguous status as a not-yet. Disability is not yet something to which a community needs to respond, at least not all the time." Whereas provision of care for older populations is positioned as an urgent and complex policy crisis (with good reasons), the provision of support for adults with disabilities is perpetually deferred as "not yet" important.

More nuanced conversations about care shift from discussion of the rote availability of services to questions of quality, human resources, and training. Personal support workers (PSWs) provide the majority of hands-on support in long-term care, which in policy conversations encompasses residential long-term care homes, private retirement homes, nonprofit and for-profit home care agencies, and sometimes the range of available attendant services. There are high turnover rates and ongoing worker shortages in PSW positions, even in challenging economic contexts (Denton et al. 2006). This inconsistent workforce also has inconsistent education, with an array of educational programs in private, public, online, and even school board settings. To take stock, there are not enough PSWs, they do not stay in their jobs, they are required to work in multiple settings with an expanding client base that has increasingly complex needs, and there are ongoing concerns about the quality and variability of the training options available to them. This indeed sounds like the making of a crisis.

Independent Living attendants, with or without any formal training, can be lumped into discussions about the complex long-term care landscape without awareness of the unique Independent Living perspective and history. This chapter insists that attendant services be considered as part of the crisis of care in ways that do not subsume the uniqueness of adulthood with physical disability or contribute to "alarmist demography" that positions disabled people as problems (Katz 1992). Current discussions of a crisis of care maintain disability within the "not-yet" time described by Titchkosky (2011), where research, attention, and policy on aging and care are urgently important (which they are) but disability is "not yet" a priority. This chapter considers the potential of "now" instead of "not yet" for direct funding, attendant services, and disability in Ontario.

Governments in the Global North are scrambling to pilot and implement new strategies to address this crisis of care. In Ontario, this includes a decision against regulating PSWs (HPRAC 2006), an ambiguous implementation of a PSW registry (Laporte and Rudoler 2013), with phased-in registration requirements for PSWs employed in varied sectors; development of new legislation, including the 2007 Long-Term Care Act and the 2010 Retirement Homes Act; and, in 2014, the release of a common education standard to be applied to all programs that train PSWs (Kelly and Bourgeault 2015). In 2014, the provincial budget also announced a wage increase for PSWs (Sousa 2014), though this increase initially excluded attendants working under Direct Funding, another example of how setting attendant services apart from other forms of care can have unintended consequences. At the same time, the closure and subsequent class-action settlement related to abuse in the Ontario regional centres and the development of a new Transformation policy framework for addressing people with intellectual and developmental disabilities signifies the enduring legacy of deinstitutionalization and perhaps early evidence of a shift related to models of care that will be socially tolerated.

Direct funding is frequently cited as one possible solution to these issues, a solution that is strongly endorsed by Independent Living movements. Indeed, the 2014 Ontario budget commits to exploring self-directed options for seniors, and Direct Payments are already available to seniors and other groups in the United Kingdom (Sousa 2014). Despite the potential to "solve" certain aspects of the care crisis and endorsement by disability advocates, this policy approach raises questions about how our practices and conceptualizations of care are transformed as Canadians increasingly enact neoliberal agendas in daily life. Amid the flurry of advocacy and program implementation, direct-funding models change the daily experience of support in complex ways and transform our understandings of care. Direct funding dramatically alters the working conditions for attendants and leaves many other oppressive practices of care unaddressed, and the insistence that "we do not need care" perhaps represents a relic in evolving disability movements. When care for older people is of such an urgent concern, there are effects of removing care and controlling its meanings in parallel conversations about Independent Living attendant services.

Strategic Removal

The Ontario Self-Managed Attendant Services' Direct Funding Program includes strong messages rejecting care, thus entering into public and theoretical rhetoric about the care crisis. Yet, a few self-managers, attendants, and informal supports demonstrated that not everyone *cares* about the term "care." For example, consider this exchange between me and Theresa, an informal support to one of the self-managers:

> CK: I've gotten some very angry reactions. Like some people just hate the word "care," they feel it's so offensive almost, but some people just ...
> Theresa: But that's what you're doing.
> CK: Well I ... I don't know.
> Theresa: I don't get that.
> CK: Well, it's the medical and the kind of charitable history of the term ...
> Theresa: Yeah ... I have no problem with that term at all. It doesn't anger me at all. I use it all the time. And that's what they're doing. I mean they are, they are taking care of [him]. You know they feed him, they toilet him, they put him to bed. Like, that's what you do when you care and you're their caregiver.

In parallel, self-manager Nick comments, "I think I prefer 'services.' But ... it doesn't bother me either way." For some people in this study, debates on care have become an issue of semantics. It can indeed appear to be the case when one only considers the messages conveyed through formal documentation for the Direct Funding Program. The less-visible picture includes defining what care is, with many far-reaching implications. It can be difficult to see the entire process, even for those who are deeply engaged in the community or related academic literature. The sense of "not caring about care" also reveals political and cultural strategies for the anti-care messages within disability movements that may not be reflected by individual attendants or self-managers. Other evidence shows a strategic element – most significantly, changes in the discourse when referring to people with intellectual disabilities. That is, although care does not happen under Direct Funding because it is primarily an oppressive outlook on disability (so the message goes), it is not exclusively an oppressive outlook. If care is a tension, as I argue in this book, the oppressive potentials of care may be transferred to other groups of disabled and older people. The participants reserve care for those who need support making decisions and, at the same time, do not condone the social exclusion of people with intellectual disabilities. Further, although the anti-care messages seem soundly anti-medical at times, various leaders concede to funding under the Ministry of Health and Long-Term Care in Ontario, again indicating a strategic function to the rhetoric. The rejection of care not only is a strategy for challenging cultural conceptions of disability but also a strategy for changing the way attendant services are delivered and experienced, among other ramifications.

Removing care complicates and nuances public rhetoric about the crisis of care. Independent Living attendant services are set apart from other types of care and demographics. Attendant services serve as an intervention and valuable counterpoint in policy and academic discussions about care, though this counterpoint is not always present in policy documents, conferences, and media stories about long-term care in Ontario. Even in my first conversation with Killian, it was apparent that the crisis of care is much more layered than simply the availability of services. Using examples from our early conversation, I now explore the removal of care in the context of a broader care crisis.

Individual Crisis of Care Caused by System Failures

Messages about care in the Direct Funding Program remind us that the crisis of care is not an abstract policy issue but difficult and challenging individual experiences that occur on a regular basis. Certainly, self-managers experience feelings of empowerment, increased flexibility, and control in their daily lives as a result of the Direct Funding Program. Highlighting the oppressive potentials of care is a reminder of the constant risk of being stranded, excluded from the program, or not having enough attendant-service hours. Self-managers stand to benefit the most when the message is effective; unfortunately, both self-managers and attendants bear the brunt when this message is too complex to be incorporated into the policy process. For example, it is the attendants who must live out the inattention to working conditions, and self-managers who wait years on the waiting list; both will feel the effects of being an unusual perspective in policy conversations about PSWs. Self-managers and attendants are quite literally left to fend for themselves in terms of when to bend the rules, styles of management, and what types of relationships are appropriate.

In many ways, Direct Funding is the ideal program for Killian's personality and lifestyle. But even as a testament to how the program can and does work, it does not provide Killian with enough attendant-service hours to fully support him in his daily life. His place of employment provides him with additional attendant support, paid separately, during the day. We discuss:

CK: If your work didn't give you support, would you have enough hours? Because [you said earlier that] your work paid for some of your hours.

Killian: No. I would only get two hours a day [from Direct Funding].

CK: Two hours a day?

Killian: At work. Or that's what I did before. For about seven years I was alone all day.

CK: So what would you do if you had to go to the bathroom or something suddenly happened?

Killian: Someone, it only happened to me a couple of times, and a co-worker asked me what's wrong or what ... and they helped me.

Killian found himself in crisis at his place of employment, forced to develop his own solution to his bodily needs. The program, for all the benefits and appeal, does not fully "solve" Killian's individual crises of care. At another point, Killian describes a period of severe illness when he was hospitalized, and his primary concern was making sure his attendants were paid even though they were not providing his support "because they have to make a living." Killian is left with a heavy responsibility to look for attendants to work short shifts at unusual times, negotiate what he terms "awkward" relationships with them, and fill in the gaps when the program falls short by asking a co-worker or establishing rapport with attendants and drawing on this. Indeed, the most liberating aspects of Direct Funding are also the most cumbersome. Direct-funding models of support cannot be regarded as a panacea for the crisis of care in Ontario, or elsewhere, as indeed these models create individual, visceral experiences of crisis on a regular basis and are only effective for very specific demographics. Simultaneously, the programs also provide an unparalleled freedom and flexibility that is simply not available in other care settings, and help enact ongoing efforts at deinstitutionalization of disabled populations. The conundrum of using direct funding models of support is thus a perpetual need to balance vulnerability, flexibility, and choice and underscores the inherent tensions of care.

Layers of Crisis

Removing care from Independent Living attendant services highlights the role of attitudes in shaping the daily realities of those who need support and of those who work in care-related fields. The way appropriate and meaningful "care" is constituted is complex. It depends greatly on the personalities of individual workers and recipients of support and the dynamic between them, and perhaps is a rationality that cannot be taught (Waerness 1996). Providing "good care" is not a given but must be worked at, interrogated, and intentionally cultivated within two-way relationships. The crisis of care includes the urgent need to focus on attitudes of attendants, self-managers, administrators, and those who develop home care policies. Independent Living also emphasizes that support can be empowering and respectful only if the environment and policy mechanisms make room for these elements. This aspect of removing care is part of why attendants specifically like working under Direct Funding and self-managers unanimously prefer Direct Funding over other styles of service delivery. For example, Killian describes the shortcomings of another attendant arrangement he used, which also formally endorsed an Independent Living approach:

> *Killian:* [I didn't like the twenty-four-hour supported living unit because] they claim they're Independent Living, but they're not. I find they're not totally Independent Living because you have to work within the demands of the attendants and the other clients, so if you wanted to get up at nine or if there are four people who want to get up at nine and there are only three attendants working, well you can't get up at nine. So I found that pretty restrictive. And the other thing I found is that they did not hire very good people. Some of them were not very nice. Or, did they really care about their job? This one attendant, he worked there part time and he worked in a hospital as an orderly full time and he was in his forties. And he did not really talk to me. Because he had that institutionalized behaviour where you go do your work and get out of there.
>
> *CK:* So he would just come and stick you in the shower without even talking to you?
>
> *Killian:* Or cook dinner. Or he came up with another attendant and they talked all the time.
>
> *CK:* And just ignored you.
>
> *Killian:* Basically. Yeah. I felt like they were only there because they had a job to do.

In this example, the problem with "care" includes inadequate infrastructure and disrespectful attitudes of the attendants. Further, Killian wonders if the attendant really cares about his job, again making room for the concept of care within Independent Living. Removing care from Direct Funding, at least in the abstract (since the above example was also of Independent Living attendant services), helps illuminate these shortcomings and demonstrates the complexity of the crisis of care that encompasses a crisis of infrastructure and attitudes.

People with disabilities, older people, and others who require short- or long-term at-home support feel the effects of inadequate home care arrangements. Removing care from our understandings of home care also reveals the layered meanings of the crisis of care. The true crisis of care is not just about how powerful and "healthy" people will "take care of the needy," but also about whether powerful policy makers who may be disconnected from daily experiences of physical dependence can develop transformative programs and services. Our policy makers have to address how to support informal care providers, properly compensate paid attendants, and address power dynamics in individual care relationships in sustainable ways. These negotiations most often remain only possibilities, as many care infrastructures do not provide time or space to actively work on these dynamics. Killian recounts an experience where he was coerced to give a large sum of money to an attendant:

> *Killian:* And for the next couple of weeks (after I wrote the cheque), I was so mad at myself ... So a couple weeks later, I said to this guy, "Look man, I don't think this is working out. I need to let you go." And I explained my situation. He goes, "Okay, goodbye." That's it. So, basically I fired the guy ... I should have fired him before on the money issue. I should have pulled the trigger right away ... Because you know what? I didn't know what he would have done, or, because like you said, we are [a] pretty vulnerable population. And I think about that all the time.

On the surface, this is an example where there is no crisis. The hours of "care" were available, and an attendant was in place and who showed up for his shifts to support Killian. The availability of services, however, did not prevent the financial abuse, or eliminate the feelings of vulnerability, or address power relationships between the attendant and Killian. Removing care from attendant services does not eliminate vulnerabilities and dependencies but reminds us of the potential of abuse, coercion, and compassion in home care relationships and the legacy of institutionalization. Killian understands that multiple layers of power are at play in attendant relationships and articulates structural issues facing attendants:

> If you go into these twenty-four-hour attendant care buildings, if you really look at the work they do, some of it is pretty in-depth, and they have more medical procedures ... And if you're getting $12 or $13 an hour and dealing with all this, along with some client attitudes, I don't think they get paid enough at all.

Workers must be respected and fairly compensated, and must learn to cultivate "good care" practices as part of addressing the power dynamics and systematic oppression within attendant services. Removing care serves as a reminder that the availability of basic services is often not enough to fully support people with disabilities or the attendants who support them (and may even be detrimental).

Home care and attendant services are not neutral; this is not a crisis of lack and a solution of provision. Services must be developed in a manner that acknowledges the power implicit in government-funded programs and the ways in which many forms of oppression manifest in home care settings.

A Crisis for Theory?

Accessible care presumes that access is "an interpretative relation between bodies" (Titchkosky 2011, 3) that is constantly evolving; accessibility is a critical reflection on the connections between discourse, spaces, and bodies. Care can be defined only as a complex tension, one that includes the notion that it can be a form of oppression for both disabled people and people who provide support. Further, as discussions in this book show, it is clear there are arenas from which care must be removed and reinterpreted. Removing care alters the debates about care among feminist and disability scholars; it is not a matter of care versus independence, but preventing care from being a totalizing approach to disability and support. It is an attempt to complicate disability and discussions about a crisis of care by bringing different voices to the table.

The altered debate does not necessarily pose a crisis for these theoretical discussions. The process of pushing care out of attendant services but not eliminating it resonates with work on relational autonomy. Clement (1996) and Chattoo and Ahmad (2008) argue that relationships and care are not contrary to notions of autonomy but form the foundation of individuals' experience of independence. The challenge for academics, policy makers, and activists is to reveal the ways in which relationships enable autonomy. Critiques of care can be used to develop practices that are based on these more accurate definitions independence, a core cultural concept that typically serves to devalue informal and formal care, service, and many forms of gendered work. Community activist Johanna encapsulates this complex position on the changing centrality of notions of in/ter/dependence:

> Well, I'm kind of making light of it, but literally I cannot live my day without being accompanied by somebody. Or if I did live a day, then six hours of being accompanied and not the rest of it, I would live an extremely limited life. And I'm just not interested in having a limited life. So it's always been sort of to me that it's about relationship and how it can, one, justify/sustain/ make a good use of, create a valuable opportunity for two people to go through life together or multiple twos of people to go through life together so that it's possible for full participation to be there, right? In my case, me plus one of

six other people are going through my day together to live a valuable life. And it always has to be a dynamic, I can't imagine that [my attendant] sitting here beside me and beside you is really not really there, right?

Johanna critiques the six-hour limit of the Direct Funding model and the idea of "arms and legs" by acknowledging her attendants as full humans who she can't imagine ignoring, even rhetorically. Johanna and her attendants "go through life together." Johanna's unusual validation of interdependence and public admittance of dependency ("I cannot live my day without being accompanied by somebody") does not mean an abandonment of independence, or full participation. Indeed, as Johanna describes, in/ter/dependence is dynamic.

The new terms for this debate are not found exclusively in this study and can be often overlooked. For example, Connie Panzarino (1994, 119–20) writes in her autobiography, *The Me in the Mirror*:

[My friend] Tom was really great. If he saw me struggling with something I couldn't reach, or writing when my hand had gotten tired and my words were beginning to look like scrambled eggs, he would say something like "Do you need a hand? You look like you're getting tired." Sometimes I accepted the help and other times I preferred to struggle. He was fine with both.

This passage is set in the late 1960s, when Panzarino was a student at New York's Hofstra University. She endorses throughout her book a consumer-directed, Independent Living approach to attendant services, but this endorsement does not necessarily place autonomy above all other values. As in the case with Ontario's Direct Funding Program, Panzarino's adamant rejection of care and removal from attendant services does not signal a denial of interdependence but serves a broader role in reclaiming authority and challenging long-standing medical and charitable institutions. It is not a paradox for Panzarino to be dependent and independent, but a reflection of how all people live. Theoretically, it is significant that, in Panzarino's experience, care is both removed from Independent Living and transformed in the bigger picture.

Behind the Story

This study is a testament to the story behind the story: nuances and complexities are revealed in the narratives behind public documents. The lived and public narratives are not in competition, but rather serve different ends. The public messages about Direct Funding proclaim "This is not care," but the other part of this process, equally interesting and potentially transformative, is implied, made apparent only through conversations. As this exploration of the Direct Funding Program illustrates, public messages have elements of strategy and are often shaped in response to political and economic contexts or parallel initiatives in international arenas. Tying messages about disability and care to a practical, concrete solution like Direct Funding is a powerful combination resulting in substantive cultural and material effects. These include empowering changes for individuals with disabilities using the program, and altering the terms of academic conversations about care, disability, and feminism. Yet, as seen through the narratives of participants in this study, there are also unintended consequences of this framework, resonating through various public policy issues, shaping which issues are highlighted and addressed within the program itself, and appearing within disability movements in Canada.

By moving care out of attendant services but not eliminating it completely, Independent Living creates spaces and conditions for autonomy and helps position people with disabilities as active citizens. The major hurdles to accessing these promises include waiting out the long wait list, passing the interview process, finding reliable and suitable attendants, and then working within the constraints of the program, which may mean insufficient attendant-service hours. Considering the complete process of removing care makes it possible for one self-manager to say "I guess Independent Living is what takes care of me" without meaning that she, or people with disabilities, should be spoken for, managed, or abused. By moving the concept of care, Independent Living in some respects represents a deeply caring framework that treats disabled people fairly, respectfully, and as full humans. Killian explains why he does not use the word "care":

> Let's just say you are my attendant and you come in one night for dinner to help me with dinner and I say, "Oh, Chrissy, would you mind helping me out tomorrow night? Because someone can't do it." I think you would be more willing to do it than, than if I go, "Hey, Chrissy, I need care tomorrow night, would you mind working for me tomorrow night?" I try to take the institutionalized language out of everything I do.

As Killian's comment shows, it is unusual to use the first person when referring to needing or receiving care. It is uncommon to be an active participant who declares "I need care" or "I am cared for," as we are accustomed to talking about "providing care for" or "taking care of" someone else. Care is indeed steeped in myriad meanings, including oppressive ones. Efforts to move care away from

Independent Living help limit its oppressive reach in practice and academic conversations while contributing in unexpected ways to discussions among policy makers. These efforts influence daily conversations between attendants and self-managers who, through living and doing Independent Living, resist the legacies and mentalities of "caring for" while transforming the meanings of care within their relationships and beyond.

Works Cited

Abbas, Jihan, and Jijian Voronka. 2014. "Remembering Institutional Erasures: The Meaning of Histories of Disability Incarceration in Ontario." In *Disability Incarcerated: Imprisonment and Disability in the United States and Canada*, ed. Liat Ben-Moshe, Chris Chapman, and Allison C. Carey, 121–38. New York: Palgrave Macmillan. http://dx.doi.org/10.1057/9781137388476.0012.

Accessibility Standards for Customer Service. 2007. http://www.ontario.ca/laws/regulation/070429.

Adams, Gina, Monica Rohacek, and Kathleen Snyder. 2008. "Child Care Voucher Programs: Provider Experiences in Five Counties." Washington, DC: Urban Institute. http://research.urban.org/publications/411667.html.

Adams, Tracey L. 2010. "Profession: A Useful Concept for Sociological Analysis?" *Canadian Review of Sociology* 47 (1): 49–70. http://dx.doi.org/10.1111/j.1755-618X.2010.01222.x.

ADAPT Free Our People! 2010. http://www.adapt.org.

Angrosino, M.V. 2003. "L'Arche: The Phenomenology of Christian Counterculturalism." *Qualitative Inquiry* 9 (6): 934–54. http://dx.doi.org/10.1177/1077800403254810.

Arenas Conejo, Míriam. 2011. "Disabled Women and Transnational Feminisms: Shifting Boundaries and Frontiers." *Disability & Society* 26 (5): 597–609. http://dx.doi.org/10.1080/09687599.2011.589193.

Armstrong, Pat, Hugh Armstrong, Albert Bannerjee, Tamara Daly, and Marta Szebehely. 2011. "Structural Violence in Long-Term Residential Care." *Women's Health & Urban Life* 10 (1): 111–29.

Armstrong, Hugh. 2001. "Social Cohesion and Privatization in Canadian Health Care." *Canadian Journal of Law and Society/Revue Canadienne." Droit Social* 16 (2): 65–81.

Arneil, Barbara. 2009. "Disability, Self Image and Modern Political Theory." *Political Theory* 37 (2): 218–42. http://dx.doi.org/10.1177/0090591708329650.

Aronson, Jane, Margaret Denton, and Isik Zeytinoglu. 2004. "Market-Modelled Home Care in Ontario: Deteriorating Working Conditions and Dwindling Community Capacity." *Canadian Public Policy/Analyse de Politiques* 30 (1): 111–25.

Art Gallery of Ontario. 2011. "Our Compass: sprOUT Art Exhibition." http://www.ago. net/our-compass-sprout-art-exhibition.

Askheim, Ole Petter. 1999. "Personal Assistance for Disabled People: The Norwegian Experience." *International Journal of Social Welfare* 8 (2): 111–20. http://dx.doi.org/ 10.1111/1468-2397.00072.

Bach, Michael. 2009. "The Right to Legal Capacity under the UN Convention on the Rights of Persons with Disabilities: Key Concepts and Directions for Law Reform." Draft discussion paper prepared for Inclusion International. Canadian Association of Community Living.

Bach, Michael, and Melanie Rock. 1996. *Seeking Consent to Participate in Research from People Whose Ability to Make an Informed Decision Could Be Questioned: The Supported Decision-Making Model.* Toronto: Roeher Institute.

Bakan, A.B., and D. Stasiulis. 1994. "Foreign Domestic Worker Policy in Canada and the Social Boundaries of Citizenship." *Science and Society* 58 (1): 7–33.

Bannerjee, Albert. 2009. "Long-Term Care in Canada: An Overview." In *A Place to Call Home: Long-Term Care in Canada,* ed. Pat Armstrong, Madeline Boscoe, Barbara Clow, Karen Grant, Margaret Haworth-Brockman, Beth Jackson, Ann Pederson, Morgan Seeley, and Jane Springer, 29–57. Halifax: Fernwood Publishing.

Barnartt, Sharon N. 2008. "Social Movement Diffusion? The Case of Disability Protests in the US and Canada." *Disability Studies Quarterly* 28 (1). http://dsq-sds.org/article/ view/70/70.

Barnes, Colin. 2007. "Direct Payments and Their Future: An Ethical Concern?" *Ethics and Social Welfare* 1 (3): 348–54. http://dx.doi.org/10.1080/17496530701603095.

Barnes, Marian. 2006. *Caring and Social Justice.* New York: Palgrave Macmillan.

Beatty, Phillip W., Gordon W. Richmond, Sherri Tepper, and Gerben DeJong. 1998. "Personal Assistance for People with Physical Disabilities: Consumer-Direction and Satisfaction with Services." *Archives of Physical Medicine and Rehabilitation* 79 (6): 674–77. http:// dx.doi.org/10.1016/S0003-9993(98)90043-0.

Beckett, Clare. 2007. "Women, Disability, Care: Good Neighbours or Uneasy Bedfellows?" *Critical Social Policy* 27 (3): 360–80. http://dx.doi.org/10.1177/0261018307078847.

Beer, Charles. 2010. "Charting a Path Forward: Report of the Independent Review of the Accessibility for Ontarians with Disabilities Act, 2005." http://www.mcss.gov.on.ca/en/ mcss/publications/accessibility/charles_beer/tableOfContents.aspx.

Ben-Moshe, Liat, Chris Chapman, and Allison C. Carey, eds. 2014. *Disability Incarcerated: Imprisonment and Disability in the United States and Canada.* New York: Palgrave Macmillan. http://dx.doi.org/10.1057/9781137388476.

Bensing, Jozien. 2000. "Bridging the Gap: The Separate Worlds of Evidence-Based Medicine and Patient-Centered Medicine." *Patient Education and Counseling* 39 (1): 17–25. http:// dx.doi.org/10.1016/S0738-3991(99)00087-7.

Bérubé, Michael. 1998. *Life as We Know It: A Father, a Family, and an Exceptional Child.* New York: Vintage Books.

–. 2010. "Equality, Freedom, and/or Justice for All: A Response to Martha Nussbaum." In *Cognitive Disability and Its Challenge to Moral Philosophy,* ed. Eva Feder Kittay and Licia Carlson, 97–110. Malden, MA: Wiley-Blackwell. http://dx.doi.org/10.1002/ 9781444322781.ch5.

Bhandar, Davina. 2004. "Renormalizing Citizenship and Life in Fortress North America." *Citizenship Studies* 8 (3): 261–78. http://dx.doi.org/10.1080/1362102042000256998.

Bhattacharya, Kakali. 2007. "Consenting to the Consent Form: What Are the Fixed and Fluid Understandings between the Researcher and the Researched?" *Qualitative Inquiry* 13 (8): 1095–115. http://dx.doi.org/10.1177/1077800407304421.

Bill 77 (Bill 77: Services for Persons with Developmental Disabilities Act, Legislative Assembly of Ontario, 39th Assembly, 1st Sess.). 2008.

Bill 118 (Bill 118 Accessibility for Ontarians with Disabilities Act, Legislative Assembly of Ontario, 38th Assembly, 1st Sess.). 2005.

Blyth, Craig, and Ali Gardner. 2007. "'We're Not Asking for Anything Special': Direct Payments and the Carers of Disabled Children." *Disability & Society* 22 (3): 235–49. http://dx.doi.org/10.1080/09687590701259427.

Boris, Eileen, and Jennifer Klein. 2006. "Organizing Home Care: Low-Waged Workers in the Welfare State." *Politics & Society* 34 (1): 81–108. http://dx.doi.org/10.1177/0032329205284757.

Breitkreuz, Rhonda S. 2005. "Engendering Citizenship? A Critical Feminist Analysis of Canadian Welfare-to-Work Policies and the Employment Experiences of Lone Mothers." *Journal of Sociology and Social Welfare* 32 (2): 147–65.

Brodie, Janine. 2008. "Putting Gender Back In: Women and Social Policy Reform in Canada." In *Gendering the Nation-State: Canadian and Comparative Perspectives*, ed. Yasmeen Abu-Laban, 165–84. Vancouver: UBC Press.

Buch, Elana D., and Karen M. Staller. 2007. "The Feminist Practice of Ethnography." In *Feminist Research Practice*, ed. Sharlene Nagy Hesse-Biber and Patricia Lina Leavy, 187–221. Thousand Oaks, CA: Sage. http://dx.doi.org/10.4135/9781412984270.n7.

Calacare. 2013. "First-in-Canada, CalaCare Combines Home Care Services with Consumer Technology." Press release. http://www.newswire.ca/en/story/1214123/first-in-canada -calacare-combines-home-care-services-with-consumer-technology.

Caldwell, Joseph, and Tamar Heller. 2003. "Management of Respite and Personal Assistance Services in a Consumer-Directed Family Support Programme." *Journal of Intellectual Disability Research* 47 (4–5): 352–67. http://dx.doi.org/10.1046/j.1365-2788.2003.00496.x.

–. 2007. "Longitudinal Outcomes of a Consumer-Directed Program Supporting Adults with Developmental Disabilities and Their Families." *Intellectual and Developmental Disabilities* 45 (3): 161–73. http://dx.doi.org/10.1352/1934-9556(2007)45[161:LOOACP]2. 0.CO;2.

Campbell, Jane, and Mike Oliver. 1996. *Disability Politics: Understanding Our Past, Changing Our Future*. London: Routledge.

Canada Revenue Agency. 2011. "Factors that Will Prevent an Organization from Being Registered as a Charity." http://www.cra-arc.gc.ca.

Canadian Association for Community Living, and People First of Canada. 2011. "Institution Watch." http://www.institutionwatch.ca/.

Canadian Council on Social Development. 2004. "Persons with Disabilities and Health." CCSD's Disability Information Sheet, no. 14. www.ccsd.ca/images/research/ DisabilityResearchPDF/drip14.pdf.

Card, Claudia. 1990. "Caring and Evil." *Hypatia* 5 (1): 101–8. http://dx.doi.org/10.1111/ j.1527-2001.1990.tb00393.x.

Carey, Allison C., and Lucy Gu. 2014. "Walking the Line between Past and Future: Parents' Resistance and Commitment to Institutionalization." In *Disability Incarcerated: Imprisonment and Disability in the United States and Canada*, ed. Liat Ben-Moshe, Chris Chapman, and Allison C. Carey, 101–20. New York: Palgrave Macmillan. http://dx.doi. org/10.1057/9781137388476.0011.

Carmichael, Angie, and Louise Brown. 2002. "The Future Challenge for Direct Payments." *Disability & Society* 17 (7): 797–808. http://dx.doi.org/10.1080/0968759022000039082.

Carnoy, Martin. 1998. "National Voucher Plans in Chile and Sweden: Did Privatization Reforms Make for Better Education?" *Comparative Education Review* 42 (3): 309–37. http://dx.doi.org/10.1086/447510.

Carroll, William K. 1997. "Social Movements and Counterhegemony: Canadian Contexts and Social Theories." In *Organizing Dissent*, ed. William Carroll, 3–38. Toronto: Garamond Press.

CBC News. 2008. "Wiseman Says No to Full Government Control of Home-Care Industry." http://www.cbc.ca/news/canada/newfoundland-labrador/wiseman-says-no-to-full -government-control-of-home-care-industry-1.741440.

–. 2010. "G20 Protester Claims Police Took Prosthetic Leg." http://www.cbc.ca/news/canada/ toronto/g20-protester-claims-police-took-prosthetic-leg-1.903985.

–. 2011. "Ontario Won't Regulate Personal Care Workers." http://www.cbc.ca/news/canada/ toronto/ontario-won-t-regulate-personal-care-workers-1.907601.

Chapman, Chris. 2012. "Colonialism, Disability, and Possible Lives: The Residential Treatment of Children Whose Parents Survived Indian Residential Schools." *Journal of Progressive Human Services* 23 (2): 127–58. http://dx.doi.org/10.1080/10428232.2012. 666727.

Chappell, Bill. 2011. "Occupy Wall Street: From a Blog Post to a Movement." National Public Radio News. http://www.npr.org/2011/10/20/141530025/occupy-wall-street -from-a-blog-post-to-a-movement.

Charlton, James I. 1998. *Nothing about Us without Us: Disability Oppression and Empower-ment.* Berkeley: University of California Press. http://dx.doi.org/10.1525/california/ 9780520207950.001.0001.

Chattoo, Sangeeta, and Waqar I.U. Ahmad. 2008. "The Moral Economy of Selfhood and Caring: Negotiating Boundaries of Personal Care as Embodied Moral Practice." *Sociology of Health & Illness* 30 (4): 550–64. http://dx.doi.org/10.1111/j.1467-9566.2007.01072.x.

Chivers, Sally. 2007. "Barrier by Barrier: The Canadian Disability Movement and the Fight for Equal Rights." In *Group Politics and Social Movements in Canada*, ed. Miriam Smith, 307–28. Peterborough, ON: Broadview Press.

Christensen, Karen. 2010. "Caring about Independent Lives." *Disability & Society* 25 (2): 241–52. http://dx.doi.org/10.1080/09687590903537562.

Church, Kathryn, Timothy Diamond, and Jiji Voronka. 2004. *In Profile: Personal Support Workers in Canada.* Toronto: RBC Institute for Disability Studies Research and Edu-cation, Ryerson University.

CILT (Centre for Independent Living in Toronto). 2000. *Direct Funding General Information.* 4th ed. Toronto: CILT.

–. 2008. *Financial Administration Start-Up Package for Self-Managers and Bookkeepers: Self-Managed Attendant Services-Direct Funding Program.* 3rd ed. Toronto: CILT.

–. 2010. http://www.cilt.ca/default.aspx.

–. 2012. "Integration of the Direct Funding Program with the LHIN System." *The Self Manager* 3-4 (Winter 2012). http://www.cilt.ca/Documents%20of%20the%20CILT%20 Website/SM-2011Winter.pdf

–. 2014. "Funding Increase Will Help More Ontarians with Disabilities Live Independently." CILT News Release. http://cilt.operitel.net/Documents%20of%20the%20CILT%20 Website/DF2014exp.pdf.

Clare, Eli. 1999. *Exile & Pride: Disability, Queerness, and Liberation.* Cambridge, MA: South End Press.

Clement, Grace. 1996. *Care, Autonomy, and Justice: Feminism and the Ethic of Care.* Boulder, CA: Westview Press.

–.Ottawa Event, hosted by the Raise the Rates Campaign. Ottawa. May 7, 2014.

Cobble, Dorothy Sue, and Michael Merrill. 2008. "The Promise of Service Worker Unionism." In *Service Work: Critical Perspectives,* ed. Marek Korczynski and Cameron Lynne Macdonald, 153–74. New York: Routledge.

Collins, Patricia Hill. 2009. *Black Feminist Thought: Knowledge, Consciousness and the Politics of Empowerment.* New York: Routledge Classics. First published 1990.

Community Living Ontario. 2009. "Deinstitutionalization." http://www.communityliving ontario.ca.

Corker, Mairian. 1999. "Differences, Conflations and Foundations: The Limits to 'Accurate' Theoretical Representation of Disabled People's Experience?" *Disability & Society* 14 (5): 627–42. http://dx.doi.org/10.1080/09687599925984.

Cranford, Cynthia J. 2005. "From Precarious Workers to Unionized Employees and Back Again? The Challenges of Organizing Personal-Care Workers in Ontario." In *Self-Employed Workers Organize: Law, Policy and Unions,* ed. Cynthia J. Cranford, Judy Fudge, Eric Tucker, and Leah F. Vosko, 96–135. Montreal: McGill-Queen's University Press.

Crawford Class Action Services. 2014. "Regional Centre Class Actions." http://huronia classaction.com/.

Cruess, Richard L., and Sylvia R. Cruess. 2006. "Teaching Professionalism: General Principles." *Medical Teacher* 28 (3): 205–8. http://dx.doi.org/10.1080/01421590600643653.

Cushing, Pamela, and Tanya Lewis. 2002. "Negotiating Mutuality and Agency in Care-Giving Relationships with Women with Intellectual Disabilities." *Hypatia* 17 (3): 173–93. http://dx.doi.org/10.1111/j.1527-2001.2002.tb00946.x.

CWDO (Citizens with Disabilities – Ontario). 2011. http://cwdo.org/d/.

Daly, Mary. 2002. "Care as a Good for Social Policy." *Journal of Social Policy* 31 (2): 251–70. http://dx.doi.org/10.1017/S0047279401006572.

DAMN 2025. 2008. damn2025.blogspot.ca/.

Davis, Courtney B., Carol B. Cornman, Marcia J. Lane, and Maria Patton. 2005. "Person-Centered Planning Training for Consumer-Directed Care for the Elderly and Disabled." *Care Management Journals* 6 (3): 122–30. http://dx.doi.org/10.1891/cmaj.6.3.122.

Davis, Ken. 1993. "On the Movement." In *Disabling Barriers-Enabling Environments,* ed. J. Swain, Vic Finkelstein, Sally French, and Mike Oliver, 285–92. London: Sage.

Davis, Lennard J. 1995. *Enforcing Normalcy: Disability, Deafness, and the Body.* New York: Verso.

–. 2002. *Bending over Backwards: Disability, Dismodernism & Other Difficult Positions.* New York: New York University Press.

Deal, Mark. 2003. "Disabled People's Attitudes toward Other Impairment Groups: A Hierarchy of Impairments." *Disability & Society* 18 (7): 897–910. http://dx.doi.org/10. 1080/0968759032000127317.

DeJong, Gerben. 1983. "Defining and Implementing the Independent Living Concept." In *Independent Living for Physically Disabled People,* ed. Nancy Crewe and Irving Zola, 4–27. San Francisco: Josey-Bass.

DePoy, Elizabeth, and Stephen Gilson. 2004. *Rethinking Disability: Principles for Professional and Social Change.* Pacific Grove, CA: Brooks/Cole.

Dick, Bob. 2009. "Action Research Literature 2006–2008: Themes and Trends." *Action Research* 7 (4): 423–41. http://dx.doi.org/10.1177/1476750309350701.

Disabled People against Cuts (DPAC). 2014. dpac.uk.net.

Dobrowolsky, Alexandra. 2008. "Interrogating 'Invisibilization' and 'Instrumentalization': Women and Current Citizenship Trends in Canada." *Citizenship Studies* 12 (5): 465–79. http://dx.doi.org/10.1080/13621020802337832.

Doucet, Andrea. 2006. *Do Men Mother? Fathering, Care, and Domestic Responsibility*. Toronto: University of Toronto Press.

Denton, Margaret, I.U. Zeytinoglu, S. Davies, and D. Hunter. 2006. "The Impact of Implementing Managed Competition on Home Care Workers' Turnover Decisions." *Healthcare Policy* 1 (4): 106–23.

Douglas, Patty. 2010a. "The Paradox of 'Care': Disability Studies' Challenge." Paper presented at the annual meeting of the Society for Disability Studies. Philadelphia, June 2–5, 2010.

–. 2010b. "'Problematising' Inclusion: Education and the Question of Autism." *Pedagogy, Culture & Society* 18 (2): 105–21. http://dx.doi.org/10.1080/14681366.2010.488039.

Driedger, Diane. 1989. *The Last Civil Rights Movement: Disabled People's International*. New York: St. Martin's Press.

Driedger, Diane, and Michelle Owen. 2008. "Introduction." In *Dissonant Disabilities: Women with Chronic Illnesses Explore Their Lives*, ed. Diane Driedger and Michelle Owen, 1–16. Toronto: Canadian Scholars' Press and Women's Press.

Duffy, Mignon. 2005. "Reproducing Labor Inequalities: Challenges for Feminists Conceptualizing Care at the Intersections of Gender, Race, and Class." *Gender & Society* 19 (1): 66–82. http://dx.doi.org/10.1177/0891243204269499.

Eady, Piers. 2014. "Independent Living Fund: Government to Close Vital Lifeline for the Severely Disabled." *Mirror*, March 7, 2014. Accessed April 29, 2014. http://www.mirror.co.uk/news/uk-news/independent-living-fund-government-close-3215627.

Earle, Sarah. 1999. "Facilitated Sex and the Concept of Sexual Need: Disabled Students and Their Personal Assistants." *Disability & Society* 14 (3): 309–23.

Ellis, Carolyn. 2007. "Telling Secrets, Revealing Lives." *Qualitative Inquiry* 13 (1): 3–29. http://dx.doi.org/10.1177/1077800406294947.

Encalada, Evelyn, Erika Del Carmen Fuchs, and Adriana Paz. 2008. "Migrant Workers under Harper: 'Guests,' Servants and Criminals." In *The Harper Record*, ed. Teresa Healy, 197–204. Ottawa: Canadian Centre for Policy Alternatives.

England, Kim. 2010. "Home, Work and the Shifting Geographies of Care." *Ethics Place and Environment* 13 (2): 131–50. http://dx.doi.org/10.1080/13668791003778826.

Engster, Daniel. 2007. *The Heart of Justice: Care Ethics and Political Theory*. New York: Oxford University Press. http://dx.doi.org/10.1093/acprof:oso/9780199214358.001.0001.

Erevelles, Nirmala. 2006. "Disability in the New World Order." In *Color of Violence: The Incite! Anthology*, ed. Incite! Women of Color against Violence, 25–31. Cambridge, MA: South End Press.

–. 2011. *Disability and Difference in Global Contexts: Enabling a Transformative Body Politic*. New York: Palgrave Macmillan. http://dx.doi.org/10.1057/9781137001184.

–. 2014. "Thinking with Disability Studies." *Disability Studies Quarterly* 34 (2). http://dsq-sds.org/article/view/4248/3587.

Erickson, Loree. 2007. "Revealing Femmegimp: A Sex-Positive Reflection on Sites of Shame as Sites of Resistance for People with Disabilities." *Atlantis* (Mount Saint Vincent University) 31 (2): 42–52.

Evans, John. 2003. *The Independent Living Movement in the UK*. http://digitalcommons.ilr. cornell.edu/cgi/viewcontent.cgi?article=1438&context=gladnetcollect.

Finch, Janet, and Dulcie Groves. 1983. *A Labour of Love: Women, Work and Caring*. Boston: Routledge and Kegan Paul.

Fine, Michelle. 1992. *Disruptive Voices: The Possibilities of Feminist Research*. Ann Arbor: University of Michigan Press.

Fine, Michelle, Lois Weis, Susan Weseen, and Loonmum Wong. 2000. "For Whom? Qualitative Research, Representations, and Social Responsibilities." In *Handbook of Qualitative Research*, ed. Norman K. Denzin and Yvonna S. Lincoln, 107–31. Thousand Oaks, CA: Sage.

Fine, Michael D. 2007. *A Caring Society? Care and Dilemmas of Human Service in the 21st Century*. New York: Palgrave Macmillan.

Fine, Michael, and Caroline Glendinning. 2005. "Dependence, Independence or Interdependence? Revisiting the Concepts of 'Care' and 'Dependency.'" *Ageing and Society* 25 (4): 601–21. http://dx.doi.org/10.1017/S0144686X05003600.

Fineman, Martha Albertson. 2004. *The Autonomy Myth: A Theory of Dependency*. New York: New Press.

Folbre, Nancy. 2006. "Nursebots to the Rescue? Immigration, Automation, and Care." *Globalizations* 3 (3): 349–60. http://dx.doi.org/10.1080/14747730600870217.

Foreign Affairs and International Trade Canada. 2009. Government of Canada Tables Convention on Rights of Persons with Disabilities. http://www.international.gc.ca/ media/aff/news-communiques/2009/368.aspx?lang=eng.

Fritsch, Kelly. 2010. "Intimate Assemblages: Disability, Intercorporeality, and the Labour of Attendant Care." *Critical Disability Discourse/Discours Critiques dans le Champ du Handicap* 2. http://cdd.journals.yorku.ca/index.php/cdd/article/viewFile/23854/ 28098.

Gardner, Julian, and Louise Glanville. 2005. "New Forms of Institutionalization in the Community." In *Deinstitutionalization and People with Intellectual Disability: In and Out of Institutions*, ed. Kelley Johnson and Ranneveig Travstadottir, 222–30. Vancouver: UBC Press.

Garland-Thomson, Rosemarie. 1997. *Freakery: Cultural of the Extraordinary Body*. New York: New York University Press.

–. 2002. "Integrating Disability, Transforming Feminist Theory." *NWSA Journal* 14 (3): 1–32. http://dx.doi.org/10.2979/NWS.2002.14.3.1.

–. 2009. *Staring: How We Look*. New York: Oxford University Press.

–. 2011. "Misfits: A Feminist Materialist Disability Concept." *Hypatia* 26 (3): 591–609. http://dx.doi.org/10.1111/j.1527-2001.2011.01206.x.

Garton, Sue, and Fiona Copland. 2010. "'I Like This Interview; I Get Cakes and Cats!': The Effect of Prior Relationships on Interview Talk." *Qualitative Research* 10 (5): 533–51. http://dx.doi.org/10.1177/1468794110375231.

Ghai, Anita. 2002. "Disability in the Indian Context: Post-Colonial Perspectives." In *Disability/Postmodernity: Embodying Disability Theory*, ed. Mairian Corker and Tom Shakespeare, 88–100. New York: Continuum.

Gibson, Barbara. 2006. "Disability, Connectivity and Transgressing the Autonomous Body." *Journal of Medical Humanities* 27 (3): 187–96. http://dx.doi.org/10.1007/s10912 -006-9017-6.

Gibson, Barbara E., Dina Brooks, Dale DeMatteo, and Audrey King. 2009. "Consumer-Directed Personal Assistance and 'Care': Perspectives of Workers and Ventilator Users." *Disability & Society* 24 (3): 317–30. http://dx.doi.org/10.1080/09687590902789487.

Gilligan, Carol. 1982. *In a Different Voice: Psychological Theory and Women's Development.* Cambridge, MA: Harvard University Press.

Glendinning, Caroline, Shirley Halliwell, Sally Jacobs, Kirstein Rummery, and Jane Tyrer. 2000. "New Kinds of Care, New Kinds of Relationships: How Purchasing Services Affects Relationship in Giving and Receiving Personal Assistance." *Health & Social Care in the Community* 8 (3): 201–11. http://dx.doi.org/10.1046/j.1365-2524.2000.00242.x.

Glenn, Evelyn Nakano. 2010. *Forced to Care: Coercion and Caregiving in America.* Cambridge, MA: Harvard University Press.

Goffman, Erving. 1961. *Asylums: Essays on the Social Situation of Mental Patients and Other Inmates.* Garden City, NY: Doubleday.

Grandey, Alicia A. 2003. "When 'The Show Must Go On': Surface Acting and Deep Acting as Determinants of Emotional Exhaustion and Peer-Rated Service Delivery." *Academy of Management Journal* 46 (1): 86–96. http://dx.doi.org/10.2307/30040678.

Grant, Karen R., Carol Amaratunga, Pat Armstrong, Madeline Boscoe, Ann Pederson, and Kay Willson. 2004. *Caring for/Caring About: Women, Home Care, and Unpaid Caregiving.* Aurora, ON: Garamond Press.

Grech, Shaun. 2011. "Recolonising Debates or Perpetuated Coloniality? Decentring the Spaces of Disability, Development and Community in the Global South." *International Journal of Inclusive Education* 15 (1): 87–100. http://dx.doi.org/10.1080/13603116.201 0.496198.

Hall, Edward. 2011. "Shopping for Support: Personalisation and the New Spaces and Relations of Commodified Care for People with Learning Disabilities." *Social & Cultural Geography* 12 (6): 589–603. http://dx.doi.org/10.1080/14649365.2011.601236.

Hall, Michael, and Keith G. Banting. 2000. "The Nonprofit Sector in Canada: An Introduction." In *The Nonprofit Sector in Canada: Roles and Relationships*, ed. Keith G. Banting, 1–28. Kingston, ON: School of Policy Studies, Queen's University.

Hamington, Maurice. 2004. *Embodied Care: Jane Addams, Maurice Merleau-Ponty and Feminist Ethics.* Chicago: University of Illinois Press.

Haraway, Donna. 1988. "Situated Knowledges: The Science Question in Feminism and the Privilege of Partial Perspective." *Feminist Studies* 14 (3): 575–99. http://dx.doi.org/10.2307/3178066.

Harrington, Mona. 2000. *Care and Equality: Inventing a New Family Politics.* New York: Routledge.

Harrison, Jane, Lesley MacGibbon, and Missy Morton. 2001. "Regimes of Trustworthiness in Qualitative Research: The Rigors of Reciprocity." *Qualitative Inquiry* 7 (3): 323–45. http://dx.doi.org/10.1177/107780040100700305.

Harvey, David. 2005. *A Brief History of Neoliberalism.* New York: Oxford University Press.

Health Canada. 2009. "Commission on the Future of Health Care in Canada: The Romanow Commission." http://www.hc-sc.gc.ca/hcs-sss/com/fed/romanow/index-eng.php.

Held, Virginia. 2005. *The Ethics of Care: Personal, Political, and Global.* New York: Oxford University Press. http://dx.doi.org/10.1093/0195180992.001.0001.

Henderson, Helen. 2007. "Join Protest If You Give a DAMN." *Toronto Star.* September 22. http://www.thestar.com/life/2007/09/22/join_protest_if_you_give_a_damn.html.

Heron, Barbara. 2007. *Desire for Development: Whiteness, Gender and the Helping Imperative.* Waterloo, ON: Wilfred Laurier University Press.

Herr, Kathryn, and Gary L. Anderson. 2005. *The Action Research Dissertation: A Guide for Students and Faculty.* Thousand Oaks, CA: Sage.

Hesse-Biber, Sharlene Nagy. 2007. "The Practice of Feminist In-Depth Interviewing." In *Feminist Research Practice*, ed. Sharlene Nagy Hesse-Biber and Patricia Lina Leavy, 110–48. Thousand Oaks, CA: Sage. http://dx.doi.org/10.4135/9781412984270.n5.

Hickson, Gerald B., James W. Pichert, Lynn E. Webb, and Steven G. Gabbe. 2007. "A Complementary Approach to Promoting Professionalism: Identifying, Measuring, and Addressing Unprofessional Behaviors." *Academic Medicine* 82 (11): 1040–48. http://dx.doi.org/10.1097/ACM.0b013e31815761ee.

Hillyer, Barbara. 1993. *Feminism and Disability.* Norman: University of Oklahoma Press.

Hochschild, Arlie Russell. 1983. *The Managed Heart: Commercialization of Human Feeling.* Berkeley: University of California Press.

–. 2000. "Global Care Chains and Emotional Surplus Value." In *On the Edge: Living with Global Capitalism*, ed. Will Hutton and Anthony Giddens, 130–46. London: Jonathan Cape.

Hondagneu-Sotelo, Pierrette. 2007. *Doméstica: Immigrant Workers Cleaning & Caring in the Shadows of Affluence.* Berkeley: University of California Press.

HPRAC (Health Professions Regulatory Advisory Council). 2006. *The Regulation of Personal Support Workers (Final Report to the Minister of Health and Long-Term Care).* Toronto: HPRAC.

Hughes, Bill, Linda McKie, Debra Hopkins, and Nick Watson. 2005. "Love's Labour Lost? Feminism, the Disabled People's Movement, and an Ethic of Care." *Sociology* 39 (2): 259–75. http://dx.doi.org/10.1177/0038038505050538.

Hutchison, Peggy, Susan Arai, Alison Pedlar, John Lord, and Colleen Whyte. 2007. "Leadership in the Canadian Consumer Disability Movement: Hopes and Challenges." *International Journal of Disability, Community & Rehabilitation* 6 (1). http://www.ijdcr.ca/VOL06_01_CAN/articles/hutchison.shtml.

Hutchison, Peggy, Susan Arai, Alison Pedlar, John Lord, and Felice Yuen. 2007. "Role of Canadian User-Led Disability Organizations in the Non-Profit Sector." *Disability & Society* 22 (7): 701–16. http://dx.doi.org/10.1080/09687590701659550.

Hwang, Hokyu, and Walter W. Powell. 2009. "The Rationalization of Charity: The Influences of Professionalism in the Nonprofit Sector." *Administrative Science Quarterly* 54 (2): 268–98. http://dx.doi.org/10.2189/asqu.2009.54.2.268.

Incite! Women of Color against Violence, ed. 2007. *The Revolution Will Not Be Funded: Beyond the Non-Profit Industrial Complex.* Cambridge, MA: South End Press.

Individualized Funding Coalition for Ontario. 2008. http://www.individualizedfunding.ca/.

Institutional Survivors. 2014. http://www.institutionalsurvivors.com/.

Integrated Accessibility Standards Regulation. 2011. August 3, 2011. http://www.ontario.ca/laws/regulation/r11191.

Jenson, Jane, and Susan D. Phillips. 2000. "Distinctive Trajectories: Homecare and the Voluntary Sector in Quebec and Ontario." In *The Nonprofit Sector in Canada: Roles and Relationships*, ed. Keith G. Banting, 29–67. Kingston, ON: School of Policy Studies, Queen's University.

Katz, Stephen. 1992. "Alarmist Demography: Power, Knowledge, and the Elderly Population." *Journal of Aging Studies* 6 (3): 203–25. http://dx.doi.org/10.1016/0890-4065(92)90001-M.

Kelly, Christine. 2010. "The Role of Mandates/Philosophies in Shaping the Interactions between Disabled People and Their Support Providers." *Disability & Society* 25 (1): 103–19. http://dx.doi.org/10.1080/09687590903363456.

–. 2011. "Making 'Care' Accessible: Personal Assistance for Disabled People and the Politics of Language." *Critical Social Policy* 31 (4): 562–82. http://dx.doi.org/10.1177/02610 18311410529.

–. 2013. "Towards Renewed Descriptions of Canadian Disability Movements: Disability Activism outside of the Non-Profit Sector." *Canadian Journal of Disability Studies* 2 (1): 1–27. http://dx.doi.org/10.15353/cjds.v2i1.68.

Kelly, Christine, and Ivy Lynn Bourgeault. 2015. "Developing a Common Education Standard for Personal Support Workers in Ontario." *Health Reform Observer – Observatoire des Réformes de Santé* 3 (1). https://escarpmentpress.org/hro-ors/article/view/169.

Kelly, Christine, and Erica Carson. 2012. "The Youth Activist Forum: Forging a Rare, Disability-Positive Space that Empowers Youth." *Journal of Youth Studies* 15 (8): 1089–106. http://dx.doi.org/10.1080/13676261.2012.693595.

Kelly, Christine, and Chris Chapman. 2015. "Adversarial Allies: Care, Harm, and Resistance in the Helping Professions." *Journal of Progressive Human Services* 26 (2): 46–66.

Kennelly, Jacqueline. 2011. *Citizen Youth: Culture, Activism, and Agency in a Neoliberal Era*. New York: Palgrave Macmillan. http://dx.doi.org/10.1057/9780230119611.

Kietzman, Kathryn G., A.E. Benjamin, and Ruth E. Matthias. 2008. "Of Family, Friends, and Strangers: Caregiving Satisfaction across Three Types of Paid Caregivers." *Home Health Care Services Quarterly* 27 (2): 100–20. http://dx.doi.org/10.1080/01621420 802022555.

Kimpson, Sally A. 2005. "Stepping Off the Road: A Narrative (of) Inquiry." In *Research as Resistance: Critical, Indigenous and Anti-Oppressive Approaches*, ed. Leslie Brown and Susan Strega, 73–96. Toronto: Canadian Scholars' Press.

King, Elizabeth M., Peter F. Orazem, and Darin Wohlgemuth. 1999. "Central Mandates and Local Incentives: The Colombia Education Voucher Program." *World Bank Economic Review* 13 (3): 467–91. http://dx.doi.org/10.1093/wber/13.3.467.

Kittay, Eva Feder. 1999. *Love's Labor: Essays on Women, Equality, and Dependency*. New York: Routledge.

–. 2002. "When Caring Is Just and Justice Is Caring: Justice and Mental Retardation." In *The Subject of Care: Feminist Perspectives on Dependency*, ed. Eva Fedar Kittay and Ellen K. Feder, 257–76. New York: Roman and Littlefield.

–. 2010. "The Personal Is Philosophical Is Political: A Philosopher and Mother of a Cognitively Disabled Person Sends Notes from the Battlefield." In *Cognitive Disability and Its Challenge to Moral Philosophy*, ed. Eva Feder Kittay and Licia Carlson, 393–413. Malden, MA: Wiley-Blackwell. http://dx.doi.org/10.1002/9781444322781.ch22.

Kittay, Eva Feder, and Licia Carlson, eds. 2010. *Cognitive Disability and Its Challenge to Moral Philosophy*. Malden, MA: Wiley-Blackwell. http://dx.doi.org/10.1002/9781 444322781.

Kohlberg, Lawrence. 1981. *Essays on Moral Development*. New York: Harper and Row.

Korczynski, Marek. 2008. "Understanding the Contradictory Lived Experience of Service Work: The Customer-Oriented Bureaucracy." In *Service Work: Critical Perspectives*, ed. Marek Korczynski and Cameron Lynne Macdonald, 73–90. New York: Routledge. http://dx.doi.org/10.4324/9780203892268.ch5.

Kroeger-Mappes, Joy. 1994. "The Ethic of Care vis-a-vis the Ethic of Rights: A Problem for Contemporary Moral Theory." *Hypatia* 9 (3): 108–31. http://dx.doi.org/10.1111/j.1527 -2001.1994.tb00452.x.

Kröger, Teppo. 2009. "Care Research and Disability Studies: Nothing in Common?" *Critical Social Policy* 29 (3): 398–420. http://dx.doi.org/10.1177/0261018309105177.

Krogh, Kari. 2004. "Redefining Homecare for Women with Disabilities: A Call for Citizenship." In *Caring for/Caring About: Women, Home Care and Unpaid Caregiving*, ed. Karen Grant, Carol Amaratunga, Pat Armstrong, Madeline Boscoe, Ann Pederson, and Kay Willson, 115–46. Aurora, ON: Garamond Press.

Lankin, Frances, and Munir A. Sheikh. 2012. "Brighter Prospects: Transforming Social Assistance in Ontario." Commission for the Review of Social Assistance in Ontario. http://www.mcss.gov.on.ca/documents/en/mcss/social/publications/social_assistance _review_final_report.pdf.

Laporte, Audrey, and David Rudoler. 2013. "Accessing Ontario's Personal Support Worker Registry." *Health Reform Observer – Observatoire des Réformes de Santé* 1 (1). https:// escarpmentpress.org/hro-ors.

Larner, Wendy. 2000. "Neo-Liberalism: Policy, Ideology, Governmentality." *Studies in Political Economy* 63 (Autumn): 5–25.

Lawson, Victoria. 2007. "Geographies of Care and Responsibility." *Annals of the Association of American Geographers* 97 (1): 1–11. http://dx.doi.org/10.1111/j.1467-8306.2007. 00520.x.

Leece, Janet. 2000. "It's a Matter of Choice: Making Direct Payments Work in Staffordshire." *Practice: Social Work in Action* 12 (4): 37–48. http://dx.doi.org/10.1080/09503150008 415197.

Levasseur, Karine. 2012. "In the Name of Charity: Institutional Support for and Resistance to Redefining the Meaning of Charity in Canada." *Canadian Public Administration* 55 (2): 181–202. http://dx.doi.org/10.1111/j.1754-7121.2012.00214.x.

Levesque, Mario. 2012. "Assessing the Ability of Disability Organizations: An Interprovincial Comparative Perspective." *Canadian Journal of Nonprofit and Social Economy Research* 3 (2): 82–103.

Lewis, Steven. 2009. "Patient-Centered Care: An Introduction to What It Is and How to Achieve It." Discussion paper for the Saskatchewan Ministry of Health. http://www. changefoundation.ca/library/patient-centred-care-an-introduction.

Lilly, Meredith B. 2008. "Medical versus Social Work-Places: Constructing and Compensating the Personal Support Worker across Health Care Settings in Ontario, Canada." *Gender, Place and Culture* 15 (3): 285–99. http://www.changefoundation.ca/library/ patient-centred-care-an-introduction.

Lindgren, Kristin. 2004. "Bodies in Trouble: Identity, Embodiment and Disability." In *Gendering Disability*, ed. Bonnie G. Smith and Beth Hutchison, 145–65. New Brunswick, NJ: Rutgers University Press.

Linton, Simi. 1998. *Claiming Disability: Knowledge and Identity*. New York: New York University Press.

Longmore, Paul K. 2003. *Why I Burned My Book and Other Essays on Disability*. Philadelphia: Temple University Press.

Lopez, Steven H. 2006. "Emotional Labor and Organized Emotional Care." *Work and Occupations* 33 (2): 133–60. http://dx.doi.org/10.1177/0730888405284567.

Lord, John. 2010. *Impact: Changing the Way We View Disability – The History, Perspective, and Vision of the Independent Living Movement in Canada*. Ottawa: Independent Living Canada.

Lugones, Maria, and Elizabeth V. Spelman. 1983. "Have We Got a Theory for You!" *Women's Studies International Forum* 6 (6): 573–81. http://dx.doi.org/10.1016/0277-5395(83)90019-5.

Lum, Janet, Jennifer Sladek, and Alvin Ying. 2010. *Ontario Personal Support Workers in Home and Community Care: CRNCC/PSNO Survey Results.* Toronto: Canadian Research Network for Care in the Community.

Lynch, Kathleen, John Baker, and Maureen Lyons. 2009. *Affective Equality: Love, Care and Injustice.* Basingstoke, UK: Palgrave Macmillan.

Lyon, Dawn, and Miriam Glucksmann. 2008. "Comparative Configurations of Care Work across Europe." *Sociology* 42 (1): 101–18. http://dx.doi.org/10.1177/0038038507084827.

Macdonald, Cameron Lynne, and David A. Merrill. 2002. "'It Shouldn't Have to Be a Trade': Recognition and Redistribution in Care Work Advocacy." *Hypatia* 17 (2): 67–83.

–. 2008. "Intersectionality in the Emotional Proletariat: A New Lens on Employment Discrimination in Service Work." In *Service Work: Critical Perspectives,* ed. Marek Korczynski and Cameron Lynne Macdonald, 113–33. New York: Routledge. http://dx.doi.org/10.4324/9780203892268.ch7.

Macleod, Rod, and Kathryn M. McPherson. 2007. "Care and Compassion: Part of Person-Centred Rehabilitation, Inappropriate Response or a Forgotten Art?" *Disability and Rehabilitation* 29 (20–21): 1589–95. http://dx.doi.org/10.1080/09638280701618729.

MacQuarrie, Anna. 2010. *Explanatory Memorandum on the United Nations Convention on the Rights of Persons with Disabilities.* Toronto: Canadian Association for Community Living.

Madrenas, Clara, and Jeff Preston. 2011. *Cripz: A Webcomic.* http://cripzthecomic.com.

Maglajlic, Rea, David Brandon, and David Given. 2000. "Making Direct Payments a Choice: A Report on the Research Findings." *Disability & Society* 15 (1): 99–113. http://dx.doi.org/10.1080/09687590025793.

Mahon, Rianne. 2008. "Varieties of Liberalism: Canadian Social Policy from the 'Golden Age' to the Present." *Social Policy and Administration* 42 (4): 342–61. http://dx.doi.org/10.1111/j.1467-9515.2008.00608.x.

Mahon, Rianne, and Fiona Robinson, eds. 2011. *Feminist Ethics and Social Policy: Towards a New Global Political Economy of Care.* Vancouver: UBC Press.

Mairs, Nancy. 1996. *Waist-High in the World: A Life among the Nondisabled.* Boston: Beacon Press.

Malacrida, Claudia. 2009. "Gendered Ironies in Home Care: Surveillance, Gender Struggles and Infantilisation." *International Journal of Inclusive Education* 13 (7): 741–52. http://dx.doi.org/10.1080/13603110903046028.

Manning, Rita C. 1992. *Speaking from the Heart: A Feminist Perspective on Ethics.* Lanham, MD: Rowman and Littlefield.

Marfisi, Carol. 2010. "Bearing the Self: A Personal Critique of Human Dynamics in PAS." Paper presented at the annual meeting of the Society for Disability Studies, Philadelphia, June 2–5.

Matthias, Ruth E., and A.E. Benjamin. 2003. "Abuse and Neglect of Clients in Agency-Based and Consumer-Directed Home Care." *Health & Social Work* 28 (3): 174–84. http://dx.doi.org/10.1093/hsw/28.3.174.

–. 2008. "Paying Friends, Family Members, or Strangers to Be Home-Based Personal Assistants: How Satisfied Are Consumers?" *Journal of Disability Policy Studies* 18 (4): 205–18. http://dx.doi.org/10.1177/1044207307311526.

Maxwell, Joseph A. 2005. *Qualitative Research Design: An Interactive Approach.* Thousand Oaks, CA: Sage.

McIntosh, Tom. 2004. "Intergovernmental Relations, Social Policy and Federal Transfers after Romanow." *Canadian Public Administration* 47 (1): 27–51. http://dx.doi.org/10.1111/j.1754-7121.2004.tb01969.x.

McRuer, Robert. 2006. *Crip Theory: Cultural Signs of Queerness and Disability.* New York: New York University Press.

Meekosha, Helen. 2011. "Decolonising Disability: Thinking and Acting Globally." *Disability and Society* 26 (6): 667–82. http://dx.doi.org/10.1080/09687599.2011.602860.

Milbern, Stacey. 2009. "Every Morning at 9 am." *Cripchick's Blog* via *Quirky Black Girls Blog.* quirkyblackgirls.blogspot.ca/2009/10/every-morning-at-9-am.html.

Millen, Dianne. 1997. "Some Methodological and Epistemological Issues Raised by Doing Feminist Research on Non-Feminist Women." *Sociological Research Online* 2 (3). http://dx.doi.org/10.5153/sro.1351.

Mingus, Mia. 2011. "Changing the Framework: Disability Justice." *Leaving Evidence.* https://leavingevidence.wordpress.com/2011/02/12/changing-the-framework-disability-justice/.

Mladenov, Teodor. 2012. "Personal Assistance for Disabled People and the Understanding of Human Being." *Critical Social Policy* 32 (2): 242–61. http://dx.doi.org/10.1177/0261018311430454.

Mohanty, Chandra Talpade. 2003. *Feminism without Borders: Decolonizing Theory, Practicing Solidarity.* Durham, NC: Duke University Press. http://dx.doi.org/10.1215/9780822384649.

Mol, Annemarie. 2006. *The Logic of Care: Health and the Problem of Patient Choice.* New York: Routledge.

Morris, Jenny. 1993. *Independent Lives? Community Care and Disabled People.* London: Macmillan.

–. 2001. "Impairment and Disability: Constructing an Ethics of Care that Promotes Human Rights." *Hypatia* 16 (4): 1–16. http://dx.doi.org/10.1111/j.1527-2001.2001.tb00750.x.

Naples, Nancy A. 2003a. *Feminism and Method: Ethnography, Discourse Analysis and Activist Research.* New York: Routledge.

–. 2003b. "Standpoint Epistemology: Explicating Multiple Dimensions." Chap. 5 in *Feminism and Method: Ethnography, Discourse Analysis, and Activist Research.* New York: Routledge.

Neufeldt, Aldred H. 2003. "Growth and Evolution of Disability Advocacy in Canada." In *Making Equality: History of Advocacy and Persons with Disabilities in Canada,* ed. Deborah Stienstra and Aileen Wight-Felske, 11–32. Concord, ON: Captus Press.

Neysmith, Sheila M., and Jane Aronson. 1997. "Working Conditions in Home Care: Negotiating Race and Class Boundaries in Gendered Work." *International Journal of Health Services* 27 (3): 479–99. http://dx.doi.org/10.2190/3YHC-7ET5-5022-8F6L.

Noddings, Nel. 1984. *Caring: A Feminine Approach to Ethics and Moral Education.* Berkeley: University of California Press.

–. 2006. "Caring and Social Policy." In *Socializing Care: Feminist Ethics and Public Issues,* ed. Maurice Hamington and Dorothy C. Miller, 27–48. Toronto: Rowman and Littlefield.

Nolin, JoAnn, and Janet Killackey. 2004. "Redirecting Health Care Spending: Consumer-Directed Health Care." *Nursing Economics* 22 (5): 251–53.

Norris, Holly. 2011. "American Able." http://hollynorris.ca.

OCSA (Ontario Community Support Association) and Attendant Services Advisory Committee. 2008. "Unleashing Attendant Services: Enhancing People's Potential, Reducing Wait Times in Acute and Long-Term Health Care." http://www.ocsa.on.ca.

Oliver, Mike. 1983. *Social Work with Disabled People*. Basingstoke, UK: Macmillan.

–. 1990. *The Politics of Disablement*. Basingstoke, UK: Macmillan.

Ontario Ministry of Community and Social Services. 2011. "Making Ontario Accessible." http://www.mcss.gov.on.ca/index.aspx.

–. 2013. "Settlement Reached in Huronia Class Action Lawsuit." http://www.mcss.gov.on.ca/en/mcss/programs/developmental/Huronia.aspx.

Panzarino, Connie. 1994. *The Me in the Mirror*. Seattle: Seal Press.

–. 1996. "To My Other Bodies." In *Pushing the Limits: Disabled Dykes Produce Culture*, ed. Shelley Tremain, 85–86. Toronto: Women's Press Literary.

Parker, Ian, Hazel Self, Vic Willi, and Judith O'Leary. 2000. *Power Shift*. Toronto: Centre for Independent Living Toronto.

Parks, Jennifer A. 2010. "Lifting the Burden of Women's Care Work: Should Robots Replace the 'Human Touch'?" *Hypatia* 25 (1): 100–20. http://dx.doi.org/10.1111/j.1527-2001.2009.01086.x.

Parreñas, Rhacel Salazar. 2001. *Servants of Globalization: Women, Migration, and Domestic Work*. Stanford, CA: Stanford University Press.

–. 2008. "The Globalization of Care Work." In *Service Work: Critical Perspectives*, ed. Marek Korczynski and Cameron Lynne Macdonald, 135–52. London: Routledge.

Payne, Jonathan. 2009. "Emotional Labour and Skill: A Reappraisal." *Gender, Work and Organization* 16 (3): 348–67. http://dx.doi.org/10.1111/j.1468-0432.2009.00448.x.

Peel, Nancye, Helen Bartlett, and Roderick McClure. 2004. "Healthy Ageing: How Is It Defined and Measured?" *Australasian Journal on Ageing* 23 (3): 115–19. http://dx.doi.org/10.1111/j.1741-6612.2004.00035.x.

Peters, Yvonne. 2003. "From Charity to Equality: Canadians with Disabilities Take Their Rightful Place in Canada's Constitution." In *Making Equality: History of Advocacy and Persons with Disabilities in Canada*, ed. Deborah Stienstra and Aileen Wight-Felske, 119–36. Concord, ON: Captus Press.

Phillips, Susan D. 1999. "Social Movements in Canadian Politics: Past Their Apex?" In *Canadian Politics*, ed. James Bickerton and Alain G. Gagnon, 371–91. Peterborough, ON: Broadview Press.

Pinterics, Natasha. 2001. "Riding the Feminist Waves: In with the Third?" *Canadian Women's Studies* 21 (4): 15–21.

Plouffe, Louise, and Alexandre Kalache. 2010. "Towards Global Age-Friendly Cities: Determining Urban Features that Promote Active Aging." *Journal of Urban Health* 87 (5): 733–39. http://dx.doi.org/10.1007/s11524-010-9466-0.

Portelli, Alessandro. 1991. *The Death of Luigi Trastulli, and Other Stories: Form and Meaning in Oral History*. Albany: State University of New York Press.

Preston, Jeff. 2008. "Mobilize March." http://www.jeffpreston.ca/about/about-jeff-preston/mobilize-march/.

–. 2011. "Operation: Stairbomb." https://www.facebook.com/stairbomb?sk=wall.

Price, Janet, and Margit Shildrick. 2002. "Bodies Together: Touch, Ethics and Disability." In *Disability/Postmodernity: Embodying Disability Theory*, ed. Mairian Corker and Tom Shakespeare, 62–75. New York: Continuum.

Price, Margaret. 2011. "Cripping Revolution: A Crazed Essay." Paper presented at the annual meeting of the Society for Disability Studies. San Jose, CA, June 15–18.

Prince, Michael J. 2009. "The Canadian Disability Community: Five Arenas of Social Action and Capacity." Chap. 5 in *Absent Citizens: Disability Politics and Policy in Canada*. Toronto: University of Toronto Press.

–. 2012. "Canadian Disability Activism and Political Ideas: In and between Neo-Liberalism and Social Liberalism." *Canadian Journal of Disability Studies* 1 (1): 1-34. http://dx.doi. org/10.15353/cjds.v1i1.16 Http://cjds.uwaterloo.ca/index.php/cjds.

Rajan, Doris. 2004. *Violence against Women with Disabilities.* Toronto: Roeher Institute.

Ridley, Julie, and Lyn Jones. 2003. "Direct What? The Untapped Potential of Direct Payments to Mental Health Service Users." *Disability & Society* 18 (5): 643–58. http://dx.doi.org/10.1080/0968759032000097861.

Rinaldi, Jenn, and Sam Walsh. 2011. "Forgotten Stakeholders: A Case for the Protecting Vulnerable People against Picketing Act." *YU Free Press* 3 (2). http://www.yufreepress.org/?p=1724.

Ritzer, George, and Craig D. Lair. 2008. "The Globalization of Nothing and the Outsourcing of Service Work." In *Service Work: Critical Perspectives*, ed. Marek Korczynski and Cameron Lynne Macdonald, 31–52. New York: Routledge. http://dx.doi.org/10.4324/9780203892268.ch3.

Roberts, Celia, Maggie Mort, and Christine Milligan. 2012. "Calling for Care: 'Disembodied' Work, Teleoperators and Older People Living at Home." *Sociology* 46 (3): 490–506. http://dx.doi.org/10.1177/0038038511422551.

Robinson, Fiona. 1999. *Globalizing Care: Feminist Theory, Ethics and International Relations.* Boulder, CA: Westview Press.

–. 2006. "Beyond Labour Rights: The Ethics of Care and Women's Work in the Global Economy." *International Feminist Journal of Politics* 83 (30): 21–42.

Roeher Institute. 1997. *Final Evaluation Report: Self-Managed Attendant Services in Ontario: Direct Funding Pilot Project.* Toronto: Centre for Independent Living Toronto.

Ronson, John. 2006. "Local Health Integration Networks: Will 'Made in Ontario' Work?" *Healthcare Quarterly* 9 (1): 46–49. http://dx.doi.org/10.12927/hcq.2006.17903.

Ryan, Sara, and Katherine Runswick-Cole. 2008. "Repositioning Mothers: Mothers, Disabled Children and Disability Studies." *Disability & Society* 23 (3): 199–210. http://dx.doi.org/10.1080/09687590801953937.

Saxton, Marsha, Mary Ann Curry, Laurie E. Powers, Susan Maley, Karyl Eckels, and Jacqueline Gross. 2001. "'Bring My Scooter So I Can Leave You': A Study of Disabled Women Handling Abuse by Personal Assistance Providers." *Violence against Women* 7 (4): 393–417. http://dx.doi.org/10.1177/10778010122182523.

Schalk, Sami. 2013. "Coming to Claim Crip: Disidentification with/in Disability Studies." *Disability Studies Quarterly* 33 (2). http://dsq-sds.org/article/view/3705.

Schriempf, Alexa. 2001. "(Re)fusing the Amputated Body: An Interactionist Bridge for Feminism and Disability." *Hypatia* 16 (4): 53–79. http://dx.doi.org/10.1111/j.1527-2001.2001.tb00753.x.

Sevenhuijsen, Selma. 1998. *Citizenship and the Ethics of Care: Feminists Considerations on Justice, Morality and Politics.* New York: Routledge. http://dx.doi.org/10.4324/9780203169384.

Shakespeare, Tom. 2006. *Disability Rights and Wrongs.* New York: Routledge.

Shakespeare, Tom, and Nick Watson. 2002. "The Social Model of Disability: An Outdated Ideology?" In *Exploring Theories and Expanding Methodologies.* Research in Social Science and Disability 2, 9–28. http://dx.doi.org/10.1016/S1479-3547(01)80018-X.

Shapiro, Evelyn. 2003. "The Romanow Commission Report and Home Care." *Canadian Journal on Aging/Revue canadienne du vieillissement* 22 (1): 13–17. http://dx.doi.org/10.1017/S0714980800003676.

Shotwell, Alexis. 2012. "Open Normativities: Gender, Disability, and Collective Political Change." *Signs* (Chicago) 37 (4): 989–1016. http://dx.doi.org/10.1086/664475.

Sidani, Souraya. 2008. "Effects of Patient-Centered Care on Patient Outcomes: An Evaluation." *Research and Theory for Nursing Practice* 22 (1): 24–37. http://dx.doi.org/10.1891/0889-7182.22.1.24.

Siebers, Tobin. 2008. *Disability Theory*. Ann Arbor: University of Michigan Press.

Silvers, Anita. 1997. "Reconciling Equality to Difference: Caring (f)or Justice for People with Disabilities." In *Feminist Ethics and Social Policy*, ed. Patrice DiQuinzio and Iris Marion Young, 23–48. Indianapolis: Indiana University Press.

Slater, Jenny. 2012. "Stepping outside Normative Neoliberal Discourse: Youth and Disability Meet – The Case of Jody McIntyre." *Disability & Society* 27 (5): 723–27. http://dx.doi.org/10.1080/09687599.2012.686879.

Smith, Andrea. 2007. "Introduction: The Revolution Will Not Be Funded." In *The Revolution Will Not Be Funded: Beyond the Non-Profit Industrial Complex*, ed. Incite! Women of Color against Violence, 1–20. Cambridge, MA: South End Press.

Smith, Miriam. 2005. *A Civil Society? Collective Actors in Canadian Political Life*. Peterborough, ON: Broadview Press.

Soldatic, Karen. 2013. "The Transnational Sphere of Justice: Disability Praxis and the Politics of Impairment." *Disability & Society* 28 (6): 744–55. http://dx.doi.org/10.1080/09687599.2013.802218.

Sousa, Charles. 2014. "Ontario Budget 2014: Budget Papers." www.ontario.ca/budget.

Spalding, Karen, Jillian R. Watkins, and A. Paul Williams. 2006. *Self-Managed Care Programs in Canada: A Report to Health Canada*. http://www.hc-sc.gc.ca/hcs-sss/pubs/home-domicile/2006-self-auto/index-eng.php.

Spandler, Helen. 2004. "Friend or Foe? Towards a Critical Assessment of Direct Payments." *Critical Social Policy* 24 (2): 187–209. http://dx.doi.org/10.1177/0261018304041950.

SSAH Provincial Coalition. 2011. http://ssahcoalition.ca.

Stainton, Tim, and Steve Boyce. 2004. "'I Have Got My Life Back': Users' Experience of Direct Payments." *Disability & Society* 19 (5): 443–54. http://dx.doi.org/10.1080/0968759042000235299.

Stasiulis, Daiva. 2004. "Hybrid Citizenship and What's Left." *Citizenship Studies* 8 (3): 295–303. http://dx.doi.org/10.1080/1362102042000257014.

Stasiulis, Daiva, and Abigail B. Bakan. 1997. "Negotiating Citizenship: The Case of Foreign Domestic Workers in Canada." *Feminist Review* 57 (1): 112–39. http://dx.doi.org/10.1080/014177897339687.

Statistics Canada. 2011. *Immigrant Status and Place of Birth (38), Immigrant Status and Period of Immigration (8A), Age Groups (8), Sex (3) and Selected Demographic, Cultural, Labour Force, Educational and Income Characteristics (277), for the Total Population of Canada, Provinces, Territories, Census Metropolitan Areas and Census Agglomerations, 2006 Census – 20% Sample Data*, 2006 Census of Population. Catalogue number 97–564–XCB200600 in Statistics Canada [database online]. http://www12.statcan.gc.ca/census-recensement/2006/dp-pd/tbt/Rp-eng.cfm?LANG=E&APATH=3&DETAIL=0&DIM=0&FL=A&FREE=0&GC=0&GID=0&GK=0&GRP=1&PID=97613&PRID=0&PTYPE=88971,97154&S=0&SHOWALL=0&SUB=722&Temporal=2006&THEME=72&VID=0&VNAMEE=&VNAMEF.

Steenbergen, Candis. 2001. "Feminism and Young Women: Alive and Well and Still Kicking." *Canadian Women's Studies* 20 (4): 6–14.

Steinberg, Ronnie J., and Deborah M. Figart. 1999. "Emotional Labor since *The Managed Heart.*" *Annals of the American Academy of Political and Social Science* 561 (1): 8–26. http://dx.doi.org/10.1177/0002716299561001001.

Stienstra, Deborah. 2003. "'Listen, Really Listen, to Us': Consultation, Disabled People and Governments in Canada." In *Making Equality: History of Advocacy and Persons with Disabilities in Canada,* ed. Deborah Stienstra and Aileen Wight-Felske, 33–47. Concord, ON: Captus Press.

Stroman, Duane F. 2003. *The Disability Rights Movement: From Deinstitutionalization to Self-Determination.* Lanham, MD: University Press of America.

Taylor, Jodie. 2011. "The Intimate Insider: Negotiating the Ethics of Friendship When Doing Insider Research." *Qualitative Research* 11 (1): 3–22. http://dx.doi.org/10.1177/1468794110384447.

Thomas, Carol. 2007. *Sociologies of Disability and Illness: Contested Ideas in Disability Studies and Medical Sociology.* New York: Palgrave Macmillan.

Tillmann-Healy, Lisa. 2003. "Friendship as Method." *Qualitative Inquiry* 9 (5): 729–49. http://dx.doi.org/10.1177/1077800403254894.

Titchkosky, Tanya. 2003. *Disability, Self, and Society.* Toronto: University of Toronto Press.

–. 2011. *The Question of Access: Disability, Space, Meaning.* Toronto: University of Toronto Press.

Tronto, Joan C. 1993. *Moral Boundaries: A Political Argument for an Ethic of Care.* New York: Routledge.

–. 2013. *Caring Democracy: Markets, Equality and Justice.* New York: New York University Press.

Tumolva, Cecilia, and Darla Tomeldan. 2004. "Domestic Workers and Caregivers' Rights: The Impact of Changes to BC's Employment Standards Regulation." *Canadian Women's Studies* 23 (3/4): 153–56.

Turner-Stokes, Lynne. 2007. "Politics, Policy and Payment – Facilitators or Barriers to Person-Centred Rehabilitation?" *Disability and Rehabilitation* 29 (20–21): 1575–82. http://dx.doi.org/10.1080/09638280701618851.

Twigg, Julia. 2000. *Bathing – The Body and Community Care.* New York: Routledge. http://dx.doi.org/10.4324/9780203190876.

Ungerson, Clare, and Sue Yeandle, eds. 2007. *Cash for Care in Developed Welfare States.* New York: Palgrave Macmillan.

United Nations Enable. 2014. "Rights and Dignity of Persons with Disabilities." http://www.un.org/disabilities/.

Valentine, Fraser. 1994. *The Canadian Independent Living Movement: An Historical Overview.* Ottawa: Canadian Association of Independent Living Centres.

–. 1996. "Locating Disability: People with Disabilities, Their Movements, and the Canadian State." Master's thesis, Carleton University.

Valentine, Fraser, and Jill Vickers. 1996. "'Released from the Yoke of Paternalism and Charity': Citizenship and the Rights of Canadians with Disabilities." *International Journal of Canadian Studies* 14 (Fall): 155–77.

van Mook, Walther N.K.A., Willem S. de Grave, Valerie Wass, Helen O'Sullivan, Jan Harm Zwaveling, Lambert W. Schuwirth, and Cees P.M. van der Vleuten. 2009. "Professionalism: Evolution of the Concept." *European Journal of Internal Medicine* 20 (4): e81–e84. http://dx.doi.org/10.1016/j.ejim.2008.10.005.

Vosko, Leah F. 2000. *Temporary Work: The Gendered Rise of Precarious Employment Relationship*. Toronto: University of Toronto Press.

Waerness, Kari. 1996. "The Rationality of Caring." In *Caregiving: Readings in Knowledge, Practice, Ethics, and Politics*, ed. Suzanne Gordon, Patricia Benner, and Nel Noddings, 231–55. Philadelphia: University of Pennsylvania Press.

Warner, Mildred E., and Raymond H.J.M. Gradus. 2011. "The Consequences of Implementing a Child Care Voucher Scheme: Evidence from Australia, the Netherlands and the USA." *Social Policy and Administration* 45 (5): 569–92.

Watson, Nick. 2002. "Well, I Know This Is Going to Sound Very Strange to You, but I Don't See Myself as a Disabled Person: Identity and Disability." *Disability & Society* 17 (5): 509–27. http://dx.doi.org/10.1080/09687590220148496.

Watson, Nick, Linda McKie, Bill Hughes, Debra Hopkins, and Sue Gregory. 2004. "(Inter) Dependence, Needs and Care: The Potential for Disability and Feminist Theorists to Develop an Emancipatory Model." *Sociology* 38 (2): 331–50. http://dx.doi.org/10.1177/0038038504040867.

Wendell, Susan. 1996. *The Rejected Body: Feminist Philosophical Reflections on Disability*. New York: Routledge.

–. 1997. "Toward a Feminist Theory of Disability." In *The Disability Studies Reader*, 2nd ed., ed. Lennard J. Davis, 260–78. New York: Routledge.

Wharton, Amy S. 2009. "The Sociology of Emotional Labor." *Annual Review of Sociology* 35 (1): 147–65. http://dx.doi.org/10.1146/annurev-soc-070308-115944.

Whitlach, Carol J., and Lynn Friss Feinberg. 2006. "Family and Friends as Respite Providers." *Journal of Aging & Social Policy* 18 (3–4): 127–39.

Wiles, Janine L., Annette Leibing, Nancy Guberman, Jeanne Reeve, and Ruth E.S. Allen. 2012. "The Meaning of 'Aging in Place' to Older People." *Gerontologist* 52 (3): 357–66. http://dx.doi.org/10.1093/geront/gnr098.

Williams, Fiona. 2001. "In and beyond New Labour: Towards a New Political Ethics of Care." *Critical Social Policy* 21 (4): 467–93. http://dx.doi.org/10.1177/026101830102100405.

–. 2011. "Towards a Transnational Analysis of the Political Economy of Care." In *Feminist Ethics and Social Policy: Towards a New Global Political Economy of Care*, ed. Rianne Mahon and Fiona Robinson, 21–38. Vancouver: UBC Press.

Williams, Val, Ken Simons, Stacey Gramlich, Gordon McBride, Natasha Snelham, and Brian Myers. 2003. "Paying the Piper and Calling the Tune? The Relationship between Parents and Direct Payments for People with Intellectual Disabilities." *Journal of Applied Research in Intellectual Disabilities* 16 (3): 219–28. http://dx.doi.org/10.1046/j.1468-3148.2003.00164.x.

Witte, John F. 2000. *The Market Approach to Education: An Analysis of America's First Voucher Program*. Princeton, NJ: Princeton University Press.

Wong, Henry D., and Richard P. Millard. 1992. "Ethical Dilemmas Encountered by Independent Living Service Providers." *Journal of Rehabilitation* 58 (4): 10–15.

World Health Organization. 2007. "Global Age-Friendly Cities: A Guide." http://www.who.int/ageing/age_friendly_cities_guide/en/.

Yoshida, Karen, Vic Willi, Ian Parker, and David Locker. 2000. *A Case Study Analysis of the Ontario Self-Managed Attendant Services Direct Funding Attendant Service Pilot: Independent Living in Action*. Toronto: Department of Physical Therapy, Faculty of Medicine, University of Toronto, in partnership with the Centre for Independent Living in Toronto.

–. 2004. "The Emergence of Self-Managed Attendant Services in Ontario: Direct Funding Pilot Project – An Independent Living Model for Canadians Requiring Attendant Services." *Research in the Sociology of Health Care* 22:177–204. http://dx.doi.org/10.1016/S0275-4959(04)22010-5.

Young, Lisa, and Joanne Everitt. 2004. *Advocacy Politics*. Vancouver: UBC Press.

Zarb, Gerry, and Pamela Nadash. 1994. *Cashing in on Independence: Comparing the Costs and Benefits of Case and Services*. London: British Council of Disabled People.

Zeytinoglu, Isik U., and Jacinta K. Muteshi. 1999. "A Critical Review of Flexible Labour: Gender, Race and Class Dimensions of Economic Restructuring." *Resources for Feminist Research* 27 (3/4): 97-121.

Zimmerman, Mary K., Jacquelyn S. Litt, and Christine E. Bose, eds. 2006. *Global Dimensions of Gender and Carework*. Stanford, CA: Stanford University Press.

Index

personal support workers (PSWs)
about, 162
as career path, 126
demographics, 126, 131, 132
global care chain, 131–32
legislation, 163
medical model and, 102
as "not care," 135
professionalization movement, 24,
100–1, 120
registry of, 134, 163
regulation of, 101, 134, 162–63
retention of, 126
training of, 100, 102, 104–5, 120, 134,
139, 162–63
wage increase for, 134, 163
See also long-term care
physical disabilities, people with
tension with intellectual disability community and, 40, 41, 43–44, 60, 110–
13, 137–38, 152–56
See also disabilities, people with
policies, government. *See* public policy
power dynamics
academic researchers and, 45–47
attendant/self-manager, 99, 168
care and oppression, 35
ethics of care literature on, 31
gender and, 77–78
in interview process, 55
medical care and, 19
in patient-centred care model, 19
physical power and, 96
risk of abuse, 78
social locations and, 38
stranding as abuse, 93–94, 98
See also oppression
Powershift (CILT), 70
Preston, Jeff, 155
Price, Janet, 57–58
Price, Margaret, 38, 58
professionalization of attendants.
See attendants, training and
professionalization
professions
definitions of, 100–1
future careers of attendants, 105, 125, 139

historical review of, 104
power dynamics and, 101, 109
redefinition of "experts," 102–4
regulation of, 100–1, 133
See also medical profession
Provincial Wait List Strategy, 12
Pruyn, John, 157–58
PSW. *See* personal support workers (PSWs)
public policy
about, 23–24, 138–40, 170–72
critiques of, 12–13
disability as a "not yet" priority, 18–19,
162
globalization of trends, 20–21
input from nonprofit organizations,
11–12, 21
ministry placement of Direct Funding
Program, 120, 135–36, 139
in neoliberal environment, 14–19
patient-centred care, 19–20
political priorities, 18–19
regulation of care workers, 24, 133–35
removal of care and discussions of,
23–24, 133
voucher systems, 19
See also activism and social justice;
direct-funding models; Direct
Funding Program; legislation; neoliberalism and austerity

queer femmegimp, 87–88

race and ethnicity
abuse of attendants, 97
attendant demographics, 20–21, 132,
139
queer women, 88
transnational subjects, 29
See also globalization and care
radical disability politics. *See* activism and
social justice
regional centres
class-action lawsuit and closure of, 4,
9–10, 97, 163
closure of, 4, 9–10
government apology for, 3–4, 10
See also institutional care

Regulated Health Professions Act, 133
relational autonomy, 33, 40, 169–70
relational work of attendants. *See* attendant services, relational work
relational work of self-managers. *See* self-managers, relational work
research in disability
  activism by researchers, 45–46, 155
  ambivalence within theories, 40–41, 43
  disability industry, 46, 47, 55, 61
  exclusion of disabled people in, 32–33
  failures in, 61
  as form of care, 52, 56
  helping imperative, 49
  neoliberal academy and, 45–46
  oppression risks, 29, 32–33, 47
  participation action research, 155
  power dynamics in, 45–47, 61
  precarious researchers, 45
  qualitative research, 22, 45, 47, 61
  reflexive process of, 61
  representation/misrepresentation in, 32–33, 46–47, 49–50, 60–61
  speaking for others, 49–50, 57–58
  structural injustices, 46
research project
  analysis of public messages, 51
  authentic times for care, 22, 91
  on care as tension, 6, 21–23, 40, 51–52
  caring relationships, 50
  data analysis, 59
  feminist perspectives on, 37
  friendship in, 55–56, 61
  impartiality in, 27
  individualized funding model and, 51
  interdependency issues, 50
  limitations of common research approaches, 32–33
  multiple perspectives in, 67
  "non-care" as concept, 22–23
  qualitative research, 6, 22, 58, 61
  representation in, 59–61
  research as form of care, 52, 56
  respondent validation, 60–61
research project, participants
  advocacy by, 145
  crises of care, 165–66
  fear of losing funding, 147–49, 165

health crises of, 106, 109–10
history of institutionalization, 3, 10, 97, 148
informal supports for, 54, 106, 122
interviews, 6, 37, 51–55, 60–61
language concerns, 54, 132
ministry placement of services for, 135–36
nonpolitical stance of, 60
postsecondary students, 126
pseudonyms, 54
recruitment of, 51, 52–54
refusal to participate, 46–47, 51, 147–48
representations in research, 46–47, 60–61
satisfaction with Direct Funding Program, 147
statistics on, 6, 51, 52
use of term "care" by, 59, 67–68, 90, 91, 163–64, 171
views on intellectual disabilities, 110–11
See also Killian and research project
research project, researcher
  autoethnography, 22, 33, 47–50, 57, 61
  former employment as attendant, 48, 49
  insider/outsider status, 56–57
  as Killian's frien-tendant, 22, 27–29
  L'Arche community experiences, 48–50
  motivation of, 48–49
  position of researcher, 27–29
  social location, 47–49, 56–57
  spouse with disabilities, 49, 54, 56
  volunteer work, 56, 155
  See also Killian and frien-tendant relationship with researcher
residential long-term care. *See* long-term care
Rideau Regional Centre, 9–10
rights-based perspectives
  on care providers, 35
  on care receivers, 19–20, 35, 39
  Charter rights, 12
  citizenship mediation, 11, 42, 105, 130
  Direct Funding Program, 9, 139–40
  Independent Living perspectives, 39
  patient-centred care, 19–20
  in public policy, 23–24

transnational issues, 42
See also UN Convention on the Rights
 of Persons with Disabilities
Roberts, Ed, 11
Robinson, Fiona, 41
Roeher Institute, 144
Rolling Quads, 11
Romanow Commission, 17, 137

sachse, jes, 155
Saxton, Martha, 94, 98, 127
Self-Managed Attendant Services, 8
See also Direct Funding Program
self-managed (home) care, as term, 7n4
See also direct-funding models
self-managers
 administrative work, 120, 148
 defined, 7, 154
 health crises, 106-7
 privacy needs, 122
 reminders of dependency, 98-99
 responsibilities, 70, 154, 166
 satisfaction with Direct Funding
  Program, 147
 training of attendants by, 102, 104-5, 133
self-managers, oppression of
 abuse risks, 97, 127
 administrative work, 120
 emergency back-up systems, 94, 120, 123
 fear of losing funding, 147-49, 165
 financial abuse of, 94-95, 168
 gender issues, 95-97
 institutionalization and, 97
 intimate personal care and, 96, 108-9
 power dynamics and, 96
 shelters for temporary protection, 95
 stranding and medical care, 109
 stranding and relational work, 23, 123
 stranding as abuse, 72-73, 93-94, 98, 99
 vulnerability if living alone, 73, 94
self-managers, relational work
 about, 88-90
 chameleon/responsive role, 86-89
 dancing metaphor for, 87
 dating metaphor for, 77
 emotional labour of, 79-83, 89-90
 empathy in, 87
 feminist studies, 84-85

institutional legacies, 4, 171
intimate personal care, 77-78, 80-82,
 85, 87, 96, 108-10
 power dynamics, 38
 social locations, 38, 85
 two-way work, 84-86, 89-90, 166
seniors. *See* older people
service industry and emotional labour,
 80-83
sexuality
 attendants and relational work, 77-78
 facilitation of sexual coupling, 87
 LGBTQ activism, 57, 155
 power dynamics, 77-78
 queer women with disabilities, 87-88
 sexual abuse, 97, 99-100, 108
 See also gender
Shildrick, Margrit, 57-58
Shotwell, Alexis, 50
Sladek, Jennifer, 126
Slater, Jenny, 158
Smith, Andrea, 141-42
social justice. *See* activism and social
 justice
social model of disability, 4n1, 10-11,
 98-99
 See also disability, as concept
social movement organizations, 141-42
 See also activism and social justice;
  nonprofit organizations
Social Services, Ministry of Community
 and. *See* Ministry of Community and
 Social Services (MCSS)
Southwestern Regional Care, 9-10
Special Services at Home (SSAH), 13, 134,
 151-52
sprOUT and LGBTQ activism, 155
SSAH. *See* Special Services at Home
 (SSAH)
supported decision-making models,
 153-54
supportive housing, 8, 167

Taylor, Jodie, 53
technology
 AODA framework and, 129-30
 attendants as assistive technology, 74-
  75, 129-31

in health settings, 74–75
reminders of dependency, 98
seniors' care, 161
temporary work permits for attendants, 21
terminology
  about, 4n1
  attendant, 7
  attendant outreach services, 8n5
  care, 90, 163–64
  consumer, 6n2, 7
  direct funding, 7
  personal assistant, 7
  self-managed (home) care, 7n4
  self-manager, 7
Thomas, Carol, 32–33
Tillmann-Healy, Lisa, 54
Titchkosky, Tanya, 18, 34, 162
Transformation initiative, 143, 150–52, 154, 163
transgender issues. *See* LGBTQ issues
transnational perspectives. *See* globalization and care
transportation issues, 130, 156
Tronto, Joan, 35, 89, 108, 115
Twigg, Julia, 80, 108

UN Convention on the Rights of Persons with Disabilities
  about, 152–54
  direct-funding models and, 142, 150
  inclusion approach, 154
  similar to a national act, 131n1
unions and Direct Funding Program, 126–27, 133
United Kingdom
  activism in, 14–15, 16, 158
  Direct Payments, 8, 15–16, 111, 149–50, 163
  disability movements, 7, 11–12
  Independent Living movement, 11–12, 16
  medical reviews and service reductions, 15n7
  neoliberalism and austerity, 14–16
  services for people with intellectual disabilities, 111, 149–50
  social model of disability, 10–11

terminology, 4n1, 7
United States
  disability justice, 143, 157
  disability movements, 7, 11–12, 141–42, 146
  Independent Living movement, 11–12
  individual vs collective advocacy, 11
  neoliberalism and austerity, 14
  terminology, 4n1, 7
universities and research. *See* research in disability
University of California, Berkeley, activism, 11

Veterans Independence Program, 7
visible minorities. *See* race and ethnicity
voucher systems, 19

Waerness, Kari, 30, 84
Watson, Nick, 114
Wendell, Susan, 33
Williams, Fiona, 31, 41–42
women. *See* gender; LGBTQ issues; sexuality
women and gendered work
  about, 29–30, 35–36, 161
  carer citizens, 113
  demographics, 131n2
  emotional labour, 79–81
  family care labour, 35
  feminist studies on, 29–30, 35–36, 69
  home settings and exploitation, 124–25
  informal supports and, 35, 39
  low wages, 35
  neglect of issues of, 29
  oppression in, 35, 114–15
  personal support workers, 126
  racialized subjects, 29, 35, 131
  transnational subjects, 20–21, 29–30, 131–32

Ying, Alvin, 126
Yoshida, Karen, 50
Youth Activist Forum, 24, 142, 155–57, 159

Zeytinoglu, Isik, 17